ETHICS AND ECONOMICS
OF HEALTH CARE

DEDICATION

For Nurses Everywhere

*They provide the majority of health care
but seldom receive the credit for it.*

ETHICS AND ECONOMICS
OF HEALTH CARE

By

GEORGE M. HALL

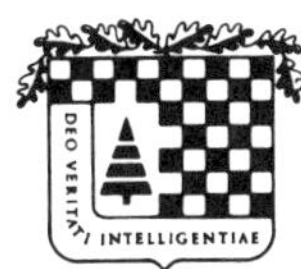

WARREN H. GREEN, Inc.
St Louis, Missouri, USA

Published by
WARREN H. GREEN, INC.
8356 Olive Boulevard
Saint Louis Missouri 63132 U.S.A.

ISBN No. 87527-495-1

Printed in the United States of America

PREFACE

This is a short book on a tall subject. It's tall because health care consumes nearly 13 percent of the gross domestic product, a percentage that continues to rise. It is short because tomes are not well read. Its preparation, however, goes back 20 years. In the early 1970's, I worked in hospital administration for five years. This included a private hospital and a medical college. The problems that are now brewing on the front pages of newspapers had already become entrenched at the time, but the magnitudes were small enough to keep them on the back burner. Still I sensed that they would eventually come to a boil and followed their progress, if that is what it may be called, ever since.

Then about a year ago I started to write this book as a discussion on the irreconcilable conflicts that underwrote the dilemma, which in turn led to the question: what do you do about it. How does one reconcile the ethics and the economics of health care, a problem that reduces to providing more care for more people at lower costs. Fortunately, I was also working on a followup to an earlier book, *Systems, Strategy and Integration*. That book explained why integrations of existing computer systems failed, wasting millions and sometimes billions of dollars.

In the process of writing it, however, I began to sense the application of the findings to systems in general and included some of that discourse within the opening chapter and again in an appendix. Then as I wrestled with the subject of health care, the ideas on systems osmosed into this book. Complex systems are complex because their internal lines of communication and transactions are complex. If that complexity stems from unnecessary or outmoded ways of doing business, that part can be streamlined, but if they are inherent in the goals of the system, then streamlining is out of the question. The key is to identify the outmoded and unnecessary lines and leave the others alone.

Still, logic and politics are two different animals, and health care has become something of a political football. It should not be surprising, therefore, that the book ends on a pessimistic note, although I have been wrong and unnecessarily pessimistic before. Once while travelling for research on another book, I had to drive long distances for the better part of two nights in a row. Upon arriving at the second destination, I went into the only eatery still open. But just as I drove up, a black Chrysler Imperial pulled up along side and four men in raincoats got out, right from the pages of Damon Runyan except there wasn't a trace of a smile on any of them. I waited in the background until they picked up their order. A few moments later, there was a commotion off to the side.

Expecting the worst I looked over in that direction with some anxiety. They were a barbershop quartet on the way back from a performance and had decided to give the late night customers a little free entertainment.

I would hope my pessimism on the score of health care proves to be equally unfounded. But I don't think it is. For example, after this book was typeset, Dr. George D. Lundberg, the editor-in-chief of American Medical Association publications, wrote a startling editorial predicting that the cost of the health care system in the United States would mushroom to $1.5 trillion dollars by 1996 and thus trigger a "meltdown" that could panic Congress into nationalizing it. This doesn't represent the official position of the AMA, but the simple fact that it was published at all in the *Journal of the American Medical Association* is indicative of its being potentially close to the truth.

Closer to home, I can see why. For example, Mutual of Omaha announced that it was raising its health insurance rates, at least for the policy I was holding, by approximately thirty-five percent. Costs are going up, but in the absence of published detailed statistics that kind of increase gives a prima facie appearance of "milking the system" for all it's worth before it finally collapses. Then I changed the policy for an agreed-upon price. When it was delivered, that price was higher than agreed to. The explanation was that the representative had made "an honest mistake" but that I, rather than the company would have to eat it up. When I disagreed with this position, the response was a curt "take it or leave it." Given that approach, Lundberg's prognosis seems conservative indeed.

* * *

I wish to express my appreciation to Polin P. Lei, a reference librarian at the Health Sciences Library at the University of Arizona. Her assistance was invaluable and she went the extra mile by making copies of pertinent articles that she came across between my visits to the library. I also wish to thank Dr. Marvin Weisbard, MD, a personal friend, for his invaluable comments in reviewing the manuscript.

CONTENTS

ETHICS AND ECONOMICS
OF HEALTH CARE

1

THE ARGUMENT

For every complex problem, there is a neat,
simple solution. And it is always wrong.
- Harry L. Mencken

Who is to say that magic and sorcery are not a part of mainstream America. A country that has accumulated a monumental debt and trade deficit, that has tolerated fraud and corruption within its own government and failed to deal with it in a timely way in the commercial banking arena, that has an all but defunct public education system, and that seems incapable of containing the illegal drug trade, is now going to create an efficient health care system at affordable rates in the middle of a major recession and rising unemployment.

Nevertheless, the lack of or at least the unaffordability of health care is slowly approaching crisis proportions. The cost is nearly 13 percent of the gross domestic product and rising. Some 35 million Americans go without health insurance and an equal number have less than adequate coverage.[1] Clearly, something must be done.

To meet the need, at least 20 different bills have been introduced in Congress. All of them subsidize health insurance to some extent but none address the roots of the accelerating cost. Further, the current administration is opposed to any form of national health insurance beyond tax credits for the indigent.[2] So the delay of controls and the emphasis on pumping more money into the system can only intensify the underlying problems. Still, this delay provides an opportunity to develop a more methodical approach instead of waiting for the haphazard solution of a government acting in a crisis later. This book addresses that opportunity.

ROOTS

For the most part the roots of the current situation in health care stem from the admirable progress in medical research and technology combined with external influences beyond the control of providers. In turn, both of these are superimposed over a traditional infrastructure that can no longer cope with the side effects. Fraud, malpractice, and administrative incompetence also take their toll, but even if these negatives were eliminated, the problem would persist.

Why medical technology is the primary root is plain. The diseases common to childhood have largely been eliminated or brought under control, and those that primarily affect individuals in their working years have at least abated. Thus the proportion of the population over 65 steadily increases. Unfortunately, the diseases and other medical conditions associated with older citizens are less amenable to cure, and moreover, the intensity and cost of that care tend to increase. The aging process taxes the ability of the body to recover, sooner or later at the 100 percent rate.

The cost of caring for the elderly is sustained to a large degree by Medicare, which when combined with the ethos of the practice of medicine, make up the second root. That ethic is to preserve life and to do no harm. For the elderly, that implementation costs a great deal of money. And as the government pays for it, or at least the majority of it, doctors do not hesitate to use extraordinary measures to preserve life at any cost.

The table illustrates the effect of these roots (costs which have risen considerably in the two subsequent years):[3]

Health Care Costs (in millions)			**Percent of GDP**	
Year	Total	Medicare	Total	Medicare
1970	$74,400	$7,633 (10.3%)	7.3%	.7%
1980	249,100	$37,533 (15.1%)	9.1%	1.4%
1989	$604,100	$240,818 (39.9%)	11.6%	4.6%

As mentioned, much of this growth stems from the infrastructure of health care financing. Hospitals and physicians lack the constraints imposed by genuine competition, while the nature of the profession weighs strongly against any further movement in that direction. At the same time, the idea of converting the existing system into a huge government monopoly is repugnant at best.

To this must be added the general decline in ethics and individual responsibility. The effect is direct in a few cases, for example "granny dumping" at emergency rooms, but it is more prevalent in the continuance of habits known to contribute to medical problems, among them: smoking, alcohol, drugs, obesity, and promiscuous sex. This is followed by an increasing demand that the government pay for the consequences as a right, the traditional sense of personal responsibility having long faded from the foreground.

Yet another root is the growing awareness that health goes far beyond the hospital and the physician's office. It encompasses diet, housing to some extent, the environment in general, education, and a host of other items. Whatever the truth or rather the extent of this may be, it is not a matter of petty cash. Food stamps alone cost the government approximately $20.3 billion a year.[4]

In any event, while the supply—the providers—may have exceeded the demand 50 years ago, just the opposite has become true in recent times. Thus the tendency has been to increase the funding to cover the differential, notwithstanding the huge federal debt and the recession. The consequence is that the magnitude of the problem compounds and makes health care even more unaffordable except for those heavily insured or subsidized.

THE NATURE OF SYSTEMS

Given the present situation and its intractable roots, the only hope lay in some sort of practical system. Unfortunately, while the provision of health care may be considered to be a system, it is one that is infinitely complex, far more so than, say, weather or ecology. To put the case another way, systems are not necessarily systematic nor can they be made so.

Science is just now coming to grip with this complex subject under the rubric of chaos[5] Nature, it seems, operates by bringing order out of chaos but at other times producing chaos and catastrophe by making minor changes to what is orderly. Perhaps the best example operates in genetics. A handful of plentiful elements combine into a cell that itself is programmed to generate an entire organism. The chromosomes remain the same in each replicated cell, but operate in specialized ways to produce differentiated cells and organs. Yet minor changes to a single cell can start it on a path of devouring its host, of which cancer is the most prevalent case.

This book is no place to delve into the intricacies of systems theory, but four points are worth noting. They are: (1) the power curve, (2) centers of gravity, often called focal points, (3) interior lines, and (4) the law of averages. These concepts are abstract but they are essential to resolving problems in anything as complex as health care.

The first of them—the power curve—is one of those concepts that everybody understands but may be hard pressed to define. When used in management and politics, it means to ride the tide of events to success, or missing that to realize that success comes only with an uphill struggle if at all. Shakespeare put that thought into *Julius Caesar*.[6] Lee Iacocca made the same point in his autobiography.[7]

The power curve operates as shown in figure 1-1. In looking at that curve, consider the effect of most pharmaceuticals. An insufficient dose (relative to the drug, the patient, and the condition) will do little good. Then once a certain threshold level is reached, the beneficial effect takes place and usually increases significantly with a slight increase to dosage. But after a certain point, any further increase in dosage has little additional benefit—the point of diminishing returns. And further increases beyond that are usually toxic and perhaps fatal.

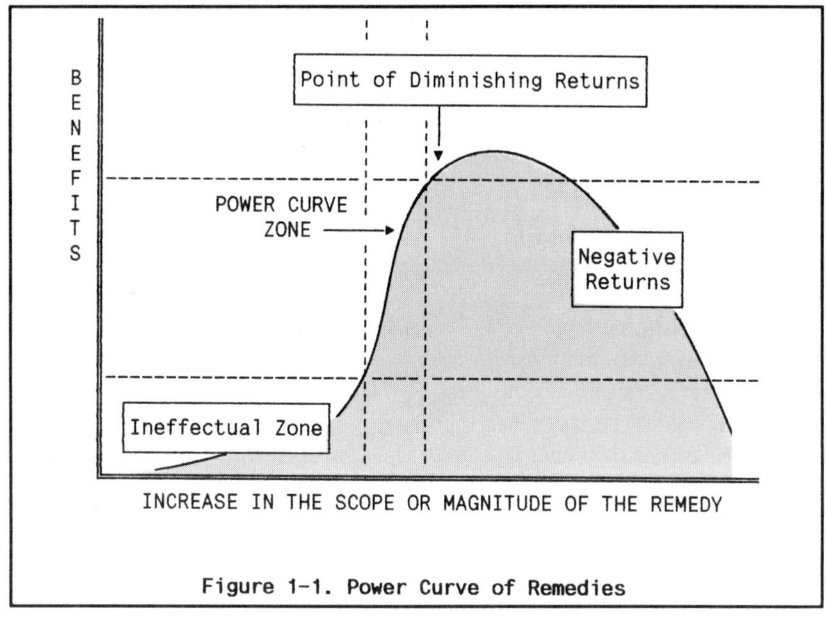

Figure 1-1. Power Curve of Remedies

The shape of this curve for any situation or system depends on many factors, but applied to health care it should be obvious that merely increasing insurance, except for those severely deprived, would be counterproductive. The accelerating costs and decreasing coverage are a classic case of diminishing returns. Moreover, the steady increase in life expectancy over the last century seems to have leveled off. Thus enormous funds are now invested on those nearing death in order to stretch out nature's process for a few months, perhaps a year, and most of that in agony. In short, at least some aspects of the current system must be revised if the power curve is to be harnessed.

The second item—centers of gravity—arises from a law in physics that states the mass of any physical object can be considered to be concentrated at a single point. For example, the ease or difficulty by which a vehicle is likely to overturn depends on the height of its center of gravity from the ground with respect to the width of that vehicle. A tall moving van is much more likely to overturn on a sharp curve than a flat-bed trailer.

Applied to human endeavors, this means identifying or creating centers of gravity so that the appropriate leverage can be applied to keep the system from toppling, or if the intent is to topple it, to do so with relative ease. Perhaps the best known example of the latter occurred during the

Battle of Midway in World War II. Six months into that war, the Japanese fleet was still the numerical superior of the U.S. counterpart, and the center of gravity for naval operations had become the carrier. Admiral Spruance, the naval task force commander, avoided a head-on sea battle and instead concentrated on sinking the four Japanese fleet carriers under the command of Admiral Yamamoto. He succeeded, leaving the Japanese only two elsewhere, and in the process turned the tide of the war against Japan earlier than anyone expected.[8]

The practice of medicine itself abounds with examples both positive or negative. Most diseases and other dysfunctions are diagnosed by recognizing the critical symptoms and hence their underlying cause, although a single condition can sometimes trigger many others. As a corollary, nothing more frustrates a physician than a patient who complains of a vague problem with equally vague and transient symptoms. True, there are a few bona fide maladies that start out like this, but more often than not it is a psychosomatic disorder or psychological need for attention.

All of this leads to the question whether the existing health care system has identifiable "centers of gravity"? The argument of this book is that it does, but they are divided into ethical and economic centers. At present, those centers do not coincide, or at least not sufficiently to bring costs under control hence improve the provision of services. They must be nudged closer together to do that, which leads to the third concept—interior lines.

This concept means the ease or difficulty with which resources, information, or anything for that matter, can be brought to bear on a problem or task. Interstate highways are an obvious example. Less than 10 percent of the U.S. highway mileage carries 90 percent of the interstate commercial traffic. This is because most of it flows among a relatively few urban areas, which, to anchor this concept to the previous one, are commercial centers of gravity.

The origin of this term comes from military science. The advantage accruing to a defender is that he has "interior lines" with which to shift his resources to meet an attacker regardless of the direction of the attack. Thus the Union forces defeated the superior Confederate forces at Gettysburg by staying entrenched on Seminary Ridge. And during the early days of the Korean war, the U.N. forces on the Pusan perimeter held out against 10-to-1 odds.

A more fascinating example is the Winchester house in San Jose, California. Sarah Winchester, who inherited the Winchester arms fortune, was told by a psychic that she would live forever if she just kept building a mansion. Surely no carpenters union ever had a better spokesman. At any rate, the mansion included stairways, hallways, and doors that lead nowhere, to confuse, so goes the story, any spirits that might otherwise do her harm. Yet beneath this facade, she designed the house to keep tabs on her servants with ease and summon them quickly to the various rooms she often occupied. This is emphasized by the tour guides, and although they don't use the term per se it is an outstanding example of imposing interior lines in what is otherwise a confusing "system." Needless to say, health care providers have not followed suit.

One last point here. Efficient interior lines are not always advantageous. Absolute monarchs and dictators may control the interior lines of their countries, but this almost always leads to disaster. Hence constitutional democracies intentionally break up those lines with "checks and balances." The idea is to check authoritarianism without snuffing out efficient government. In practice, of course, such governments are typically more inefficient than intended except in crises when the checks and balances abate somewhat in order to meet the current challenge. This is the history of the United States writ large.

So the challenge in health care is to develop the necessary lines to control costs without imposing authoritarianism. The latter means micromanagement, standardized protocols ("cookbook medicine"), and a federal auditor the constant companion of every provider. One way to avoid this, while still creating effective interior lines, is to depend on the "law of averages." This "law" states that while no one event can be predicted, a class of like events will adhere to a predictable distribution curve with distressing conformity. The most common applications are actuarial tables developed by insurance companies. In medicine, the counterpart is the Medicare disease-related group (DRGs) set of formulas for reimbursement to hospitals.

The problem with DRGs is that patients are often sent home too early in order to increase hospital revenue. The reimbursement for a specific condition (there are 442 of them in the DRG table) is the same regardless of the length of stay, therefore it "pays" hospitals to discharge patients as soon as possible. Worse, this has lead to underutilization of hospitals and so they "compete" for more patients even though such inpatient care may not always be necessary.

This, then, brings the argument to its crux: can an inefficient system be made more efficient by increasing the use of techniques that already have or can generate harmful side effects? The answer is yes, but the approach involves trade-offs. The key trade-off reinvigorates the exercise of professional judgment—one of the ethical centers of gravity—among providers in return for their accepting some strictures at critical economic centers of gravity.

APPROACH

The approach is developed in the thirteen remaining chapters. Chapter 2 reviews the bidding on 23 factors that affect health care. Would that there were fewer to consider, but health care doesn't work that way. These factors are divided into quantitative and subjective categories and are supported by two appendixes. The first (A) discusses the consequences of the expanding federal debt and the second (B) is a brief discussion of some of the negative aspects encountered in foreign health care systems.

Chapter 3 then turns to the debate between ethics and economics. The ideal is for ethics to influence economics more than the other way around, but experience suggests this is seldom the case, not only in health care but in virtually all other human endeavors. For even when ethics supposedly hold sway, what is provided must be paid for, and therein lies the inexorable force of economics.

This is followed by a chapter that more closely examines the ethical centers of gravity for health care. Conceptually, they are simple: define health care and then divide the responsibilities between providers and recipients. This is easier said than done, and because the definition will likely exceed the available funding under the best of circumstances, some form of rationing—the euphemism is limitations—will prove inevitable. Now rationing is not a pleasant word. It connotes a denial of necessary help, a practice acceptable only under emergency conditions. But if the demand for services outpaces the supply of funds under the best of circumstances, rationing would be unavoidable. [†]

Chapter 5 follows this with a more detailed look at the economic centers of gravity. For health care they are: hospital and physician reimbursement, excess hospital capacity, and the effects of proportioning the funding among taxes, premiums, copayments, and deductibles. Recipients must foot the bill in one way or another; there isn't anyone else to pick up the tab. But the idea is to strike a balance that makes health care affordable with sufficient incentives to avoid milking the system.

With those points in mind, chapter 6 presents a strawman concept for realigning the interior lines of health care management and financing. The core of it is to eliminate excess hospital capacity and then reimburse hospitals on a per diem, not a per case basis, from a singular source of national health care funding (plus recipient copayments). In addition, physician fees would be capped at reasonable levels. Any hospital that had a physician on its staff who insisted on supplementary fees for covered services would not be reimbursed. Then once the costs are throttled, the remaining problems can be dealt with piecemeal, primarily by the providers themselves and not by an intrusive government or insurance agency.

[†] The writer does not advocate rationing. The proposal merely recognizes the inevitability and then harps on checks and balances to insure those decisions are made as democratically as possible.

Chapter 7 discusses the different types of ancillary services, some of which are considered orthodox and others alternative medicine. The latter are often shunned by the former. In some cases, there is too much evidence to warrant this attitude; in others, the practices are one step removed from pure quackery. But if a national health plan is established, then it would be imperative to decide which of these ancillaries to include and which to exclude.

The next chapter addresses mental health, because that subject ranges from expensive and intensive hospital care to the high success rate of no-cost support groups. Hence in no other aspect of health care is the definition so elusive, and it also confronts the issue of personal responsibility much more sharply. In a worse case scenario, a broad definition of mental health could lead to absolute socialism.

The next two categories of issues are the emotional-laden ones and those related to automation, covered respectively by chapters 9 and 10. It is true that all issues in health care come packaged with emotional overtones, but when those overtones appear to dominate the scene, the issues must be resolved politically. That is the price of living in a democracy. And as for automation, the issues are far more important—and insidious—than commonly assumed.

Chapter 11 then reviews the advantages and disadvantages of the proposal in terms of the various infrastructures that are the main players in the present system. Anything that is new will inevitably run against the grain of the established way of doing business. In this case, as costs must be reduced, one or more parties must lose out to one degree or another. This will be resisted, even when the trade-offs are favorable.

This leads to chapter 12 on organization and responsibilities. The proposed mechanics are not necessarily the most efficient, but the political process and the influence of the existing infrastructures must be taken into account. And so there would be a three-tier organization to ensure that adequate checks and balances reside in the system. The upper tier would be a singular agency at the national level with limited but critical powers. The second level would comprise state insurance agencies for the actual management of the system, but again with relatively limited powers that would be far less intrusive on specific professional judgments. The remaining level, of course, would be the providers and the recipients themselves.

Chapter 13 outlines a dynamic model for experimenting with the various parameters and factors for a period of two years. It would be supported by a computer system that is also described briefly in the chapter. The reasoning is that the only hope of success lies in involving the existing infrastructure from the beginning but continuously confronting it with the economic consequences of its ethical leanings, and vice versa.

The last chapter then reconsiders the proposal from a higher perspective and concludes that even under the best of circumstances, neither this nor any plan that aims at reform stands much of chance for implementation. On the other hand, the mounting national debt must perforce eventually lead to a depression, especially if Congress simply throws more money at the existing health care system. At that point, the proposal or some variation on it might stand a better chance of being adopted.

* * *

A word about statistical data. Literally tons of it can be found in the literature, and therefore to sample it fairly would have doubled the length of this book. However, much of that data exists in segmented form and begs what is sometimes called *meta-analysis*. Unfortunately, that term sounds too much like metaphysics, but in reality the practice is scientific in nature and has already been applied in medical research with outstanding results. For example, the various findings from experiments and research in the treatment of some cancers has been meta-analyzed to suggest how to improve the survival rate, with startling results. Synonyms for this type of analysis include syntheses and integrated studies.

So the book deals with this problem in two ways. First, it minimizes reporting statistical data, concentrating instead on the various centers of gravity and relying primarily on orthodox sources, e.g., the American Medical Association and the Department of Health and Human Services for the data it does cite. Second, to compensate, it recommends eight integrated studies (in appendix C). Each should be pursued independently by two or more agencies. These kinds of surveys are somewhat subjective, which may be overcome in part by comparing several independent findings.

2

FACTORS

Reality exerts its own logic and overrides legal arrangements.
                                        - Hans Morganthau

Every problem is embedded in one or more factors and any attempt to deal with it must come to grips with them. Further, some of those factors may be more resistant to change or modification than others, so that difference is important too. In any event, each factor bears its own significance, hence the obligation is to make the most of that significance rather than ignore it. Else, as Hans Morganthau so wisely observed, it will return to haunt the planners.

For the purposes of this book, the factors affecting health care have been divided into quantitative and subjective categories. The former by definition are based on data and are less prone to debate, although their significance and malleability are often open questions. The latter, by contrast, are inherently more difficult to prove in any direct sense of that word. Still, ample evidence exists to warrant their inclusion here, and many of them are subjects for the proposed integrated studies outlined in appendix C.

So far so good. Unfortunately, there are 23 of these factors. This appears to go against the grain of developing a solution based on a few centers of gravity, but that is not quite the case. Complex systems are complex precisely because of the large number of factors operating within them. Reshaping that type of system—bringing some order out of its chaos—depends on finding a few critical vantage points about which the discordant factors can be viewed, linked, and managed.

QUANTITATIVE FACTORS

1. *As noted, health care costs per individual are the highest among those over 65, and the percentage of those individuals is increasing.* The significance is that the present Medicare program may be a better starting base for national health insurance than standardizing the coverage, costs, and payment of many

commercial insurers, as many as six of whom may be supporting the same hospital. In any event, the interior lines would be infinitely simpler.

2. *Excess hospital capacity is the single most malleable factor affecting health care costs.* The occupancy rate has dropped from 78% in 1972 to 69.6% in 1988.[1] The significance is that any reform should eliminate most of those excess beds and put the rest in "mothballs." Further, it should also be recognized that some of the beds that are utilized are questionable at best, spurred on by a system that tries to fill as many empty beds as possible. That "slack" can absorb temporary bona fide overflow.

3. *Physician income is rising with hospital costs, and many doctors charge more than Medicare and other government plans are willing to pay, or refuse to accept such patients at all.* Between the 1970's and 1990, physician income rose from approximately $58,000 to about $157,000.[2] Further, because so many physicians have leveled high surcharges on Medicare patients above the ceilings, Congress passed a law that as of 1992 this excess charge could be no more than 20 percent.[3] Under a national system, all surcharges would be intolerable for covered services.

4. *Physician specialties are inadequately distributed, resulting in an excess of the more highly paid specialties and a shortage of family physicians (although some remarkable strides are being made to change this).* If there were more family practitioners, there would likely be fewer hospitalizations and more minor medical problems taken care of. Specialists are hospital oriented.

5. *Fraud and malpractice are widespread but except in flagrant cases both are difficult to identify hence reduce.* The uncertain data suggests the need for a comprehensive survey, but regardless of the numbers this proposal cannot solve the problem directly.

6. *Some attempts to reduce or hold down costs have been effective but insufficient to stem the tide.* The DRG criteria, increased copayments, peer review, and prosecution for billions of dollars of fraudulent claims from providers have been an obvious success, but the total cost keeps rising. Something more radical is necessary.

7. *Insurance companies are withdrawing from the private and small group market, leaving only Blue Cross-Blue Shield and a few major commercial insurers to serve the group market.* Further, Medicare reimbursement is handled by contract with insurance agencies, more often than not the "Blues." Hence the insurance infrastructure for any national system will likely be a variant on this.

8. *Corporate employers are the focal point for the collection of taxes to fund national health insurance.* The Medicare tax is collected from employees as an adjunct to the Social Security (FICA) tax. Employers also pay for health care

insurance for active and retired works, including collection of the employee share. The significance is that a national health care tax would be little more than a consolidated variation on what already occurs.

9. *Under the present system, or any system that concentrates primarily on providing coverage, costs will continue to run amuck and eventually lead to some form of national economic collapse, not merely one in health care.* This is demonstrated in appendix A, but the logic is plain. The federal debt is growing exponentially. Without controls, national health care insurance will only exacerbate that growth. It might even happen with adequate controls, and so the system must have simple enough interior lines to adapt to a sudden change in national fortunes—in a word, resiliency.

SUBJECTIVE FACTORS

10. *A separate program for the indigent is no longer politically viable.* Vaguely analogous to the failure of the "separate but equal" doctrine to resolve racial problems, the attempt to provide health care for the indigent by way of the Medicaid program and tax supported public and VA hospitals has come up short, notwithstanding the tremendous accomplishments and the often remarkable charitable spirit of those who labor in this subsystem.

11. *Non-salaried physicians and non-public hospitals—which comprise the majority of providers in those categories—will not submit to nationalization, nor would that approach necessarily stem costs.* The experience in foreign countries, as discussed in appendix B, suggests why the latter is true. As for the former, one only need consider the enormous clout that would be marshaled against it by the existing infrastructure. In short, any acceptable cost control measures must leave room for individual and corporate providers.

12. *No matter how dedicated providers may be, the vast majority will tend to be self-serving towards their immediate interests.* The abstractions of the greater good over the long haul don't have the weight to offset the problems of "here and now," and providers spend most of their day wrestling with the latter. This idea was developed at length by Adam Smith in 1776 in *The Wealth of Nations.*

13. *There is, in addition, a minimum sludge-level of incompetence, arrogance, malpractice, and whatever, that no system will ever be able to reduce on a permanent basis.* Even Caesar Augustus, as absolute emperor of Rome and a man who ruled with considerable integrity, learned this lesson the hard way when at the end of his tenure he attempted to legislate the reform of human morals.

14. *Once any health care system is established, the tendency will be to add more coverage.* This almost goes without saying and is reinforced by the fact that the vast majority of individuals and organizations testifying before Congressional committees advocate increased spending not reductions.[4]

15. *Political solutions tend to be short sighted.* A solid case can be made that since most members of Congress have become entrenched in office, they will tend to vote for whatever helps them get reelected, and what many if not most voters want is financial help with here-and-now economic problems.

16. *The potential for shifting other federal spending to health care is limited, as is the margin for raising new taxes.* Defense spending may be cut, but the majority of it goes directly or indirectly to salaries and wages. Cut those, and unemployment goes up. Increased unemployment raises costs by way of more unemployment compensation and reduces revenues for the obvious reason. Raise taxes, and investments go down. The economy is not all that elastic.

17. *There are many unknowns in health care.* No one will disagree with that statement, but it does reinforce the need for resiliency in any national health care system. For example, the discovery of a vaccine that would be effective against cancer is highly unlikely, but cheaper and more effective methods to detect cancer early and hence destroy it while it is isolated are a sure bet. The system would do well to reduce any financial disincentives that might otherwise apply here.

18. *The conduct and habits of individuals in large measure contribute to health or its lack.* The research on tobacco products, alcohol, illegal drugs (and excess use of prescription drugs), overeating or poor nutrition (when alternatives are within financial reach), and a sedentary lifestyle, is just too overwhelming to deny.[5] What is in question is the extent to which each contributes to health or its lack. That warrants yet another survey, but the more significant point is that any health care system which downgrades personal responsibility is headed for trouble.

19. *Preventive medicine has limits and even when successful, excepting pre and post natal care, it will have a tendency to raise not decrease health care costs.* This may not have been true at one time, and it is hard to prove today but here is the reasoning. As the diseases and problems of the younger abate, the average age of the population increases. With that come even more medical problems and major increases to the total health care bill. This doesn't mean preventive medicine should be downgraded. Far from it, any deemphasis here would be intolerable. But it won't reduce overall costs.

20. *Ethics are by no means standardized.* There is no debate that taking a baby's life because it is deformed is heinous murder. Nor, at the other extreme, will many providers advocate a heart-lung transplant for a patient whose cancer had metastasized to his brain. Between these polemics, however, the range of opinions abounds. The significance is that if rationing proves inevitable, the decisions on what to ration, and how much, must be subject to due process in the broadest sense of that term.

21. *The federal government is not to be fully trusted as the final arbiter for the management of health care.* Actually, its not to be fully trusted in anything.

For example, the Justice Department leaped on a recent Supreme Court decision in order to waive the First Amendment for anything said or written with federal funding that it chose to prosecute.[6] To this must be added Watergate, Irangate, and all the other gates that various contractors and regulatees have erected in Washington to protect proprietary interests. The significance, of course, is that the federal government should be kept at arm's length in any health care system beyond those essential centers of gravity it must regulate by default.

22. *The crisis in health care is still a few years off.* Millions are uninsured, but most of them are young and only a relative few are confronted with major medical expenses (and some of that is subsidized at taxpayer expense). The majority of individuals are adequately covered and are relatively satisfied with that coverage and the providers they have access to. Finally, all but a tiny fraction of elderly Americans are covered by Medicare and most of them can afford a supplementary policy to pick up on the expenses that Medicare does not cover. As costs increase this will change and the affordability if not the availability of health care will become a crisis, but for the time being the situation is not serious enough to effect immediate change. The significance is that it provides a few years to work out a system, providing the inevitability of national health insurance is accepted as eventual fact.

23. *Beware the pot of gold at the beginning of the rainbow.* If health care devours 13 percent of the gross domestic product, and most of that is eventually channelled through a singular financing system, almost every crook and promoter, from organized crime to politician, will attempt to leech it. Hence the accounting of the distribution of funds must be both simple and highly publicized.

3

ETHICS VERSUS ECONOMICS

*I think that capitalism, wisely managed, can probably be made
more efficient for attaining economic ends than any alternative
system yet in sight, but that in itself is in many ways objectionable.*
- John Meynard Keynes

Some writers posit that capitalism is the bane of society and human conduct.
A few, notably Marx, Engels, and Lenin, carried the argument to the point where
it spawned a revolution that took root in many countries and prevailed for several
generations. But except for China and a few odd remnants, the experiment
proved an utter failure. And China is not doing all that well either.

The problem, of course, is that ethics, regardless of how worthy the motive,
cannot be imposed over economic realities. That may not be socially acceptable,
but it is reality. When Charles and Mary Beard discovered the economic
parameters that underwrote much of American history, their book raised a lot of
angst.[1] The mind may ponder ethics; the body politic feeds on economics.

The compromise has been an attempt to guide and manage democratic
nations by way of economic policy. Sometimes this is done by way of taxation;
sometimes, as advocated by Keynes, by manipulation of various economic
policies, e.g., interest rates. But this too has met with considerable failure and
often a resignation to economic realities. The reformation of health care will
likely prove no exception; on the contrary it may overtax the economy instead
of the other way around and ethics will once again take a back seat.

Some schools of ethics hold that what applies to individuals applies equally
to groups, organizations, and nations. Unquestionably there is some truth to this.
The law recognizes corporations as a kind of legal individual, and jurisdictions
are considered equivalent to corporations in some ways. Yet the law also
recognizes partnerships and individual responsibility. A group comprises individuals formed to deal with problems that the members acting alone cannot
accomplish or at least cannot accomplish well enough. This is sometimes called
a *social contract*, albeit many scholars deride the use of that term.

Moreover, an individual is free to choose for himself or herself what the leaders of a group or nation are not always free to choose for those whom they represent. One may opt to be a martyr or starve for some cause, or to speak out for one point of view even if it bores the rest of the world. Certainly, individual talents have little counterpart in organizations, or as one old saw puts the matter, a camel is a horse designed by a committee.

But in a group or government—at least those that are pegged at less than a totalitarian level—the managers do not have those options. For the most part, they strive for balance and compromise while at the same time trying to protect the group against external problems or solving internal ones that, as mentioned, are beyond the influence of individuals acting apart.

The strange thing about this is that economics is secondary to ethics in both perspectives except in the narrow sense of greed. For example, if an individual wants to concentrate on accumulating wealth, that is really a matter of ethics. A democracy is obliged to provide the environment to exercise that choice, providing other individuals are not defrauded in the process or denied their right to do the same. True, the person saturated with greed may pay a high price for it—loss of family or of sanity—but that only demonstrates priority of ethics over economics at the individual level.

At the group level, the same is true but the mechanics are different. The leader or leaders may try to provide for services for which there are insufficient funds. That brings about compromises, which ideally seek to provide for the greatest good for the greatest number, accompanied by various safety nets for the those who get the "leastest good" from such decisions. One only need read the Constitution and the Bill of Rights (the first ten amendments) to see this philosophy in operation.

The conflict, then, pits the aims of each individual against the perceived attempt by the group's management to create a balance. This implies that the needs of individual members do not fall into neat manageable patterns. It doesn't take much to prove that. Conflicts and corruption abound, and thus leaders are faced with dilemmas. In the absence of infinite resources and wisdom, compromises are made. The attempt is to spread the satisfaction, but the compromise itself may dilute the solution to the point where it won't work over the long haul.

So the real dilemma is to decide between a short-range compromise and a long-range one. The long-range variety will spread less satisfaction in the immediate future but in time the benefits should compensate for that. Perhaps the most dramatic case of this happened in Great Britain during World War II. The British had broken the German *enigma* code and knew, in one particular instance, that the Luftwaffe was scheduled to bomb Coventry. As this was not a normal target, Sir Winston Churchill was faced with the dilemma of alerting that area to save lives at the price of tipping the hat on having broken the code, or letting the raid proceed on the grounds that not tipping the hat would in the long run save more lives.[2]

Churchill was in no position to put the matter to a vote, and even if he could have, it's a safe bet the tally from Coventry would have differed markedly from the one in London. So of necessity he took matters into his own hands and decided on the latter course of action. Needless to say, this great and good man could never thereafter sleep easy with it.

And so it must be for any decision that involves a trade-off between short-range and long-range benefits, of which health care is a major example. A heart-lung transplant may save a life, but the money spent on one such operation could be invested instead in pre and post natal care for hundreds if not thousands of indigents. In the long run, a few children will gain a life that would otherwise have been denied them, and certainly many others would have fewer health problems as they grew up.

This is no abstraction. The state of Oregon has initiated planning for a rationing and priority system for Medicaid and other charity patients, but it has not met with universal approval.[3] There are those who believe it is the government's responsibility to find the resources to meet every need, regardless of the cost or consequences, which leads to an interesting conflict.

So, the essence of the ethic on the provision of health care can be stated as follows: to provide adequate health care at an affordable cost and subsidized that cost if necessary to accommodate all comers, and to restore each patient to full health if possible, or that failing due to the patient's condition, to come as close as possible. Many patients have this already but the indigent seldom do. One only need visit an inner city clinic to see this. On any given day, several hundred people may be waiting to see one of the doctors or nurses. Most of them are bedraggled, many have severe psychiatric disorders, few eat anything close to a proper diet whether they have the funds or not, and almost all of them have given up any hope of changing their lot in life.

It is true that most of them are eligible for Medicaid, but that program reimburses providers at such low rates that fewer and fewer doctors will accept this category of patient anymore, and those that do limit that part of their practice. Only pediatricians seem to keep the door open—as might be expected of professionals who specialize in the care of children—and even they have cut back somewhat on Medicaid patients.

At least this was the picture before the current recession began. Nowadays, with two to three times as many people out of work, that same clinic is the only resource for many of those who would prefer to work and pay their own way. And so this scene has become the focal point for all that is wrong with the economy and the with the availability and the affordability of health care.

Now turn to the reality of attempting to realize that ideal. Richard P.

Kusserow, Inspector General for the Department of Health and Human Services, has significantly reduced the immense fraud and overcharging endemic to Medicare. That success has been measured in billions of dollars, and eventually those savings could be used to pay for more care for indigents. Yet the American Medical Association took the step of asking President Bush to fire him on the grounds that his actions were intruding too far on the prerogatives of medicine.[4] Thankfully, he's still in business, but that doesn't eliminate the conflict.

The distance between these two scenes is considerable. On the one hand, the country is trying to ensure the greatest good for the greatest number within the limit of existing funding. On the other hand, some of the remedies applied have intruded upon professional prerogatives and soured the motivation of providers to do what is necessary. Yes, many providers are self-centered beyond any hint of compassion, and, yes, providing health care in the inner city can test the patience of the most altruistic doctor or nurse, but when a professional is treated as a robot by his government, nothing worthwhile is going to be accomplished. Talk to doctors in Great Britain.

So the requirement is to break down the problem and its impasses into its constituent parts and try something more efficacious than brute force management. To this end, the first step is to define what is to be provided. This is the primary ethical issue and assumes that the government is going to ensure that it is in fact provided. This means direct action rather than the reaction of carving savings out of a system that no longer works. It is a matter of setting up a list of priorities, and then aiming for as much of the list as possible within the realities of funding.

Second to quantity, then, comes quality and physical accessibility. Perhaps it should be the other way around, but if the quantity does not exist to start with, quality and distribution are moot points. Now if the government owns the system lock, stock and barrel, it can dictate distribution and hope for improved quality. Veterans Administration hospitals have amply demonstrated the ability of the government to distribute care to less enticing environments, at least more so than the private sector. The quality of care in the VA, however, is another matter, and a nationalization of private hospitals is not a realistic option. The alternative is to concentrate on economic incentives, leaving direct action to those few instances where there is no other recourse.

The bottom line to these points is: how much will the plan cost and who is going to pay for it. This, of course, is where economic reality comes into play. For the umpteenth billion time, there is no free lunch. Or breakfast. Or supper. Or health care. If there are insufficient funds, how is the balance to be obtained? What are the trade-offs? In the absence of adequate funding, how is the shortfall to be rationed. Back to ethics.

The resolution of this issue in part depends on who is held responsible for what. The more that individuals are held responsible for conduct and habits that lead to better health, or at least maintain existing health, is the extent to which the system can provide more. But the same cannot be applied to physicians, hospitals, and other providers in any direct sense. They can be held accountable for the quality of care provided. They can be criminally prosecuted for fraudulent charges. On the other hand, they can neither be maneuvered as pawns nor be expected to place themselves in a neat pattern of distribution.

That is something the system must do, and do it without treading on professional prerogatives and responsibilities. But at least the bottom line remains ethical in nature, and can stay that way if the economic consequences of rash or excessive public ambition, no matter how worthy the motive, are kept in check. Therefore, the next two chapters concentrate on the centers of gravity of ethics and economics, respectively, as a preface to thrashing out a realignment of the interior lines necessary to effect change.

4

ETHICAL CENTERS OF GRAVITY

*It is entirely easy to settle any question if only one principle
is involved. But the hang of it is that most questions, all questions
that are difficult, have a conflict of at least two principles.*
- Felix Frankfurter

The previous chapter argued that while ethical concerns should and initially do take precedence over economics, the latter asserts itself to become the arbiter of most conflicts. If that is the case, then a successful health care system should keep its ethical objectives within realistic economic bounds. In theory, this can be done by setting out ideals and then paring those down as necessary.

That would work if health care wasn't burdened with two pivotal issues. The first concerns the definition of health care itself. Until that is resolved, there is little hope of pinning down an ethical center of gravity, and in a democracy that definition is likely to arise pragmatically and change with the political winds.

The second issue, as brought up in the preceding chapter, is that of apportioning responsibility between providers and recipients. And because the bulk of the funds would pass through the hands of the government and a relative handful of insurance companies or agencies, they too must be factored into the equation.

Further, while these two issues are theoretically independent, they are linked in a practical way. That is, while the definition of health care may not be dependent on responsibility, resolving the latter issue will influence the scope of covered services.

THE NATURE OF HEALTH CARE

Perceptions on the nature of health care range from "delivery system" to an attempt by man to guide and modify the healing process inherent in all organisms, a debate that is no longer academic. If a decision is made to have universal insurance then agreement on what to cover must be reached. We do not need a domestic Vietnam. That war was fought with little attention paid to objectives and definitions, and in the end the United States expended countless billions of dollars and 58,000 lives with nothing to show for it.[1]

The "delivery system" perspective makes for tasty political hor d'oeuvres, but in truth very little health care is delivered. House calls are all but unheard of today. Rather, patients "deliver" themselves to physician's offices or are "delivered" to hospitals. They go to pharmacists to purchase prescriptions (although a few are sent through the mail). Occasionally government-funded clinics are established in neighborhoods without adequate private facilities, but health care is not the same thing as commerce.

So if the "delivery" concept, along with the elusive term "wellness," can be set aside, more rational alternatives can be considered. First among these would be the categories of care: (a) curative, (b) restorative, (c) palliative, and (d) custodial. It's an interesting approach, yet a visit to most any hospital will quickly demonstrate that the first three are too intermingled to serve as criteria. Only custodial care can be separated, and even much of that is closely associated with the practice of medicine.

A second approach is to weigh the proportional roles of the provider and the recipient. This runs headlong into the debate on responsibility. Is the drug addict or alcoholic—and there are more than twenty million of them in this country— diseased or otherwise afflicted beyond his or her capacity to cope? In that case, given the low rate of success in "curing" addicts by all means combined, the definition of health care would permeate the whole of life.

A third approach might hinge on the degree of cost or intensity of care required, cost often being correlated to intensity. This one has some utility to it on the grounds that the less expensive treatment is, the more it can be afforded out-of-pocket by all but the destitute. In practice the rise in copayments and deductibles for all forms of health care insurance is leaning heavily in this direction, but it is still too much of a shotgun approach.

This leaves the old fallback of the hospital. To the extent that health care is hospital oriented, in the broadest sense of that term, it could be considered as a part of health care, else not. Taking into account that physicians are increasingly clustered in office buildings near hospitals combined with an increasing emphasis on outpatient surgery and the like, this too warrants consideration. But it doesn't sit well with other perspectives, and further, one of the ideas behind any national health care plan would be to reduce unnecessary hospitalization.

The point is that none of these approaches can serve as a singular criterion. The reason is that the definition of health has no limit short of life in its entirety. Logically speaking, it is a bottomless pit. This is especially true for mental health. On the other hand, there would be little pressure for national health insurance if hospital and physician fees had kept in line with wages and salaries over the past twenty years. So a more pragmatic decision is likely to hover on the coverage now provided by Medicare and most group policies.

The problem, then, is to keep that definition in bounds and prevent the system from the inexorable slide into socialism, where the government takes on the responsibility for life "from womb to tomb" as the expression goes. "Hello. Congressman So-and-So? I wonder if you might intervene on my behalf. You see, it's my birthday this week and I want to eat an extra piece of cake, but my doctor has ordered me not do to this, or he will have my child taken away and given to foster parents because I would be setting a bad example for him." Far fetched? Not by much. Consider a current situation under adjudication in Syracuse, New York.

This case originated with the Onondaga County Department of Social Service. An unmarried mother, Denise Perrigo, was breast feeding her baby and became aroused by it. Worried that something was wrong, she sought advice from a community volunteer center. Actually, the phenomenon is by no means uncommon, but the volunteer referred her to the local rape crisis center. One thing led to the next. The baby was taken from her, and she was jailed for sexual abuse of a child. Eventually, a family court judge threw the case out and restored the child to her mother.[2]

But the local health police were not to be silenced. They immediately filed new sexual abuse charges because the mother had used a rectal thermometer. The case is still making its way through the courts, and at the moment the mother has been found innocent of abuse but guilty of neglect because, among other things, when she made the original phone call, she should have known it would lead to the ensuing trauma.

RATIONING AND ITS EUPHEMISMS

To continue, it would appear that any successful system will be obliged to ration health care in some form or to some degree. The typical euphemisms are limitations and excluded-services. However, there are many categories of rationing, and they all need to be explored. Figure 4-1 summarizes the text.

The most obvious and least debatable category comprises legal restrictions. Active euthanasia (as differentiated from withholding of medical treatment at the request of the patient) is homicide. Also, certain types of medical treatment and procedures are outlawed or severely restricted, for example the use of narcotics and experimental procedures considered experimental. And within the next few years, abortion may be outlawed except to save the life of the mother.

The balance is legal but not always covered, which brings up the category of exclusions. That is, any individual can elect to have the procedure done or the service provided if they have the means, or can obtain the means, to pay for it. Most cosmetic surgery comes under this heading, as do many very high cost procedures. The problem is that those who must do without raise the specter of health care as a right until they too become entitled to it. The egalitarian instinct in America is not to be underestimated.

Next comes the most controversial category: rationing by age or condition. An example of rationing by condition would be to deny extraordinary or so-called "aggressive therapy" to individuals who are terminally ill. An example of rationing by age would be to deny, or at least not cover, hemodialysis (kidney dialysis) for the elderly. Neither prevails in the United States, except in the de facto sense that few doctors would go ahead with major treatments for patients who are in the throes of death. It's a different story in other countries, especially the United Kingdom.

A less troublesome approach is rationing by time. This simply sets capacity below demand and then places elective procedures on a low priority waiting list. This deters some from even applying, and spreads the cost of those who wait patiently over time.

	Advantages	Disadvantages
	DIRECT RATIONING	
Coverage Exclusion	The simplest way to effect rationing in any plan. It affects all members equally.	Except for pure electives, the political tendency is to expand not curtail coverage.
Age Criterion	Highest savings. The elderly consume a vastly disproportionate share of health care costs.	The elderly won't accept it. Traditions in other countries were set when the elderly were few.
Condition Criterion	Second highest source of savings and less controversial if limited to terminally ill patients.	Agreement on criteria for time left to live, and the care that would qualify, is difficult.
	INDIRECT RATIONING	
Time Rationing	This is a marvelously simple, uncontroversial way to cut the cost of elective procedures.	Hospital capacity must be cut 40-45 percent. The grousing and gripping will be relentless.
Copayments and Variations	Very effective, and for all practical purposes unavoidable in any health care system.	In excess, they can be too much of a disincentive, especially those with the least income.
Parimutuel Funding	Encourages altruistic providers to hold down excess costs in order to expand services.	Very difficult to effect at the national level. Requires costly administration and accounting.

Figure 4-1. Direct versus Indirect Rationing

The last two categories are increased copayments or deductibles and parimutuel funding. The first is all but standard practice in the U.S. today and reduces costs by deterring the least necessary care. The second works by prioritizing all procedures and then covering, in a subsequent period, only those items which can be paid for from revenues collected in the current period. As mentioned, Oregon's plan for revising Medicaid works along these lines, but it seems to be impractical at the national level.

ROLE OF THE PROVIDER

Separating responsibilities between providers and recipients is not easy because the dividing line is fuzzy and it often varies with the details of similar situations. It also depends on whether health care is considered a right. If so, then by the nature of constitutional law, corresponding responsibilities demand consideration. Freedom of speech, observed Justice Oliver Wendell Holmes, does not extend to yelling "fire" (without cause) in a crowded theater.[3] Similarly, if there is to be "freedom from want of health care" responsibilities must be established. Else the Supreme Court will find itself reviewing medical records on appeal every time some plaintiff files suit because his or her doctor failed to cure an addiction that landed them in trouble.

Still, certain items fit providers regardless of how responsibilities are divided. Some of these sit squarely on the shoulders of each individual and organization licensed to practice medicine or provide services. Others are impractical to achieve at that level and can only be effected by funding incentives or legal controls. A doctor can be sued for malpractice. He cannot be sued because there are too few family practitioners working in the lower east side of New York or in the far reaches of Alaska.

The one unquestionable responsibility of individual providers is competence, the opposite of which is malpractice. Legally, if not professionally, malpractice varies from the most innocuous, harmless mistake to wanton negligence that results in the avoidable death of a patient. Newspapers are filled with these stories, and the cost of physician malpractice insurance is extremely high. Worse, various estimates have surmised that as many in one of ten procedures or treatments involves malpractice to some degree. Finally, as medical technology and knowledge increase, doctors can be found guilty of malpractice solely on the grounds of not keeping up with the latest protocol. It's a tough problem, but it seems to be as prevalent (if not more so) in government-run hospitals and clinics as in private practice.

Individual providers can also be pinioned on prices up to a point. Fraudulent claims can always be prosecuted under criminal statutes, but providing too much care, except in the most flagrant cases, is hard to prove and the defense is often to avoid a potential malpractice suit. Still, the era when physicians can elect to charge more than Medicare reimbursement may be coming to an end.[4]

The two remaining, easily defined responsibilities are clearly beyond the power and influence of individual providers to ensure: (a) distribution among specialties, types of hospitals, and so forth, and (b) physical distribution or accessibility. Granted, some socially conscious providers have made a real difference in some regions, but expecting all of them to become like Mother Teresa is asking too much of human nature. Besides, the Vatican does not have the manpower to process that many petitions for canonization. Fortunately, tremendous progress has been made by the medical profession itself to encourage more medical students to become family practitioners, a tendency which has been enhanced by a recent realignment of the Medicare physician reimbursement schedule.

As for physical distribution, the availability of national insurance would help, but the security problems of working in the inner city and the low population density common to rural and desert regions will take additional incentives to abate.

ROLE OF THE INDIVIDUAL

A century and a half ago, the individual was almost totally responsible for his or her health, and in the event of failure the appeal was largely to the gods. The practice of medicine was neanderthal, unsanitary, and except for a few procedures may have done more harm than good. Things have swung radically in the opposite direction since then, perhaps too much so, and as always there is no way an individual can prevent all or even most serious medical problems by right conduct and good habits. A few are born afflicted with medical problems so severe that they will be under continuous medical care all their lives. A few others are born with such healthy genes and live such a fortuitous life that they rarely see a doctor professionally. The remaining 98 percent fall between these polemics.

Unfortunately, the exact extent to which conduct or rather misconduct and habits contribute to a lesser state of health is subject to controversy and is in great need of a survey of existing findings (as noted in appendix C). Still, whatever those findings may prove to be, certain items need to be recognized: (a) conduct in general, (b) habits and addictions, (c) seeking timely help when symptoms appear, and (d) participating actively in treatment to the maximum extent possible.

Conduct includes reckless and drunk driving, poor eating habits, abuse of children, spouses, and older parents, inappropriate budget priorities (which can work against timely seeking of medical help) and several hundred other items that often if not always lead to medical problems. Habits and addictions are a variation on this, but there is more evidence of physiological roots or at least propensities, and the conduct usually (but not always) centers on abuse of a single type of substance.

Seeking timely help is also a serious problem, though failure here carries less opprobrium. Medical records are filled with cases where patients were aware of symptoms but delayed seeking insurance-covered competent help before the condition became fatal or at least before it could have been brought under more effective control. And those records are also filled with cases of patients that made little or no effort to participate in their own recovery, or who disregarded medical advice and thereby suffered additional consequences. This doesn't mean that a patient is suppose to assist in his or her own surgery. It does mean adhering to a prescribed regimen unless there is sound reason to believe that it would harmful.

In a few cases, extraordinary effort on the part of a patient has wrought almost miraculous results. Norman Cousins wrote a famous autobiographical book on that subject: *Anatomy of an Illness*. In fact, his attitude was so influential that he was invited to join the faculty of psychiatry at the UCLA medical college as an adjunct professor. This may be expecting too much from all patients, but it does prove that participation is an essential element in recovery and the maintenance of health.

All well and good, says the critic, but how do you enforce it? In practice, how can patients be encouraged to lead a better life style if they were severely abused as a child or made to participate in satanic rituals? When the drug-laced sot has stormed out of his house after beating his wife and raping his daughter, kills several people on the highway, and is then brought into an emergency room in critical condition, should treatment be denied? There are no easy answers to these questions, but economic incentives, targeted tax disincentives, and, when appropriate, mandatory pecuniary fines and jail terms come easily to mind

5

ECONOMIC CENTERS OF GRAVITY

Because that's where the money is.
- Willie Sutton
On being asked why he robbed banks

While funds for health care bobble in a hundred directions, there are three times when the bulk of them flow through narrow focal points: (a) insurance processing, (b) payments to hospitals and similar institutions, and (c) payments to physicians and other individual providers. This accounts for roughly 70 percent of the health care dollar.[1] True, most of this money then passes on, directly or indirectly, to other players. Physicians pay taxes, malpractice insurance, and office expenses. Hospitals pay employees and for supplies and services. They, in turn, further distribute funds, and so the money flows like fish in one of those huge donut-shaped tanks in showplace aquariums.

In the parlance of defense strategists, these narrow foci are called *choke points*. Major canals and narrow passageways, such as the Strait of Malacca bordering Indonesia, are choke points. Bottle them up, which is easy to do, and not much is going to get through, or only by time-consuming alternative routes. Narrow them, and the flow is constricted in proportion to the grip. By analogy, then, this is what is meant by economic centers of gravity. The simplest way to hold down costs is to apply a grip at the choke points *provided it does not strangle the patient*. This means that the money necessary to fund bona fide health care must continue to flow unabated. The balance can be shut off, subject only to political pressure to keep the former recipients alive on tubes.

INSURANCE PROCESSING

One of the most efficient insurance-type systems in the country is Social Security. Whatever the pitfalls of the present surplus being used to bankroll federal deficits may be, only a tiny fraction—probably less than one percent of the revenues collected—is used to pay for overhead.

The same is nearly true for Medicare administration, notwithstanding the operation is far more complex than direct distribution of monthly checks. Here, the overhead is a mere 2.3 cents on the dollar.[2] By contrast, commercial health insurance companies spend 14 times that much: 32 cents on the dollar. Even when Blue Cross-Blue Shield and the self-insured companies are added to the computations, the overhead is still six times higher. In practical terms, this excess amounts to about $13 billion. That could pay for a lot of health care and is a good example of the potential for gripping economic centers of gravity—choke points—in a healthy sort of way. If national health insurance were consolidated into Medicare, then funds would continue to flow where needed while unnecessary overhead, profits, and an extensive amount of fraud were eliminated.[3]

Now it is true that the profit motive drives the American economy and makes it possible for the country to afford expensive health care. But that care itself can no longer afford the luxury of "taxing" the public for further profits. And if the health insurance industry must bite the bullet, the same can be applied to providers when it comes to processing claims. That is, if simpler means can be found to average-out payments to providers, then the whole subculture of claims processing could be reduced by 80 percent or more. Sound too good to be true?

Consider how much money the government saved when it reduced item-by-item cost accounting for some elements of official travel. They discovered it was less expensive to reimburse flat amounts per day regardless of actual expenses. The occasional excess payment was negligible compared to the savings from cutting out the processing and auditing under the old method. An analogous application occurs in changing light bulbs in office buildings. Office managers discovered it was cheaper to ride circuit and replace overhead bulbs on a schedule, whether burned out or not, than to replace them on a call-by-call basis. Similar applications and examples can be found in almost every field of work.

HOSPITALS

Hospitals may be havens of mercy in the ethical sense, but they are at the mercy of a dozen forces beyond their control in the economic arena. This doesn't ignore the fact that some administrators are inflicted with the edifice complex; or that they gouge the system for high salaries, large staffs, and sumptuous office suites; or, for those to whom it applies, that they abuse the tax breaks for non-profit institutions. In that sense, they are almost as bad as elected officials. But hospitals do not control their own destiny. They can only react and in so doing become a nearly uncontrollable economic center of gravity.

Twelve of the forces that shape hospital finance are: (1) medical staffs, (2) Medicare reimbursement formulas, (3) the variety of commercial insurance reimbursement formulas, (4) the obligation to provide free care to one degree or another, (5) bad debt, (6) labor intensive budgets, (7) growing malpractice suits, (8) the "recommendations" of the periodic inspections by the Joint Council on the Accreditation of Hospitals, (9) increased reporting and documentation requirements, (10) simmering conflicts between physicians and nurses, (11) continual progress and advance in medical technology, and (12) the de facto need to compete for patients, which leads to a whole list of insidious subforces. This is not a complete list and doesn't even touch upon the special problems of teaching hospitals, but it will suffice for the purposes of this book.

The medical staff is the key pressure point. Everything in a hospital depends on patient load, and patients are admitted only by physicians. Because many if not most doctors are on the staff of more than one hospital, they can and do play one against the other to get what they want. In short, the hospital's real customers are doctors, not patients. Not surprisingly these "customers" are usually perceived as being right.

The next item is Medicare reimbursement, which accounts for the majority of revenue in some hospitals and for a substantial chunk in most others. However, as mentioned in previous chapters, Medicare reimbursement is based on average cost per disease-related group (indexed to regional costs). Most of the balance comes from Blue Cross-Blue Shield and commercial insurance companies. The former are gravitating towards the Medicare formula—indeed they administer most of it at the regional level—while the latter tend to be "bill payers." These "bill payers" get soaked for the unreimbursed costs incurred under Medicare and some of the "Blues." This is done by way of inflated costs for specific items and by inserting additional items or quantities in the bill in a kind of Robin Hood fraud.

Some of those excess costs stem from free care. By law in some states, hospitals must accept for treatment any individual who walks or is brought into an emergency room, at least until they are stabilized. If there is no coverage or payment, the cost is taken out of the hide of other patients, exclusive of Medicare. This too contributes to widespread excess charges for simple items, as documented recently on the television program *20-20*.[4] Bad debt also accounts for increased costs. This is no different than any other business, but it creates a vicious cycle. The more that costs increase, the more bad debts increase, which only lead to a new round of cost increases in an attempt to recoup the loss.

Unlike many businesses, however, hospitals are labor intensive, and much of that labor earns relatively high salaries, especially nurses and technicians. The reason is that nursing floors and some services must be staffed 24 hours a day, seven days a week, 365 days a year. When a nurse takes a vacation, she (95 percent are women) must be replaced for that period of time.

Next on the list comes malpractice. The popular conception is that physicians bear the brunt of malpractice, but hospitals are just as subject to it and they also pay huge malpractice premiums. Moreover, they have created elaborate systems of paperwork to supposedly reduce malpractice or at least minimize the damage when it does occur. This takes staffing and further raises costs.

More? Hospitals, like schools, are accredited, which means they must meet certain standards of operation, management, quality of service, and so forth. A single agency does this—the *Joint Council for Accreditation of Hospitals* or JCAH. Because a hospital cannot be reimbursed if it loses its accreditation, it doesn't take genius to deduce the clout exercised by the JCAH. And it always seems to come up with new ways to improve service by additional documentation and more reports, which leads to the next item.

Increased reporting requirements, and not just those recommended by the JCAH, also add to the bill. True, this isn't much different than anywhere else, but it is added to a field of endeavor that is already awash in paperwork. This ranges from medical records to patient care plans, to endless rescheduling, to claims processing. Much of this paperwork is completed by floor nurses. However, most of them are so busy during their shifts that taking scheduled time out for eating meals has become a luxury and taking breaks the source of a standing joke. So the paperwork gets done in overtime, at time-and-a-half wages, or at least with compensatory time. The latter leads to days off, which are then staffed by higher-cost agency or on-call (PRN) nurses.

A more subtle problem arises from the simmering conflicts between nurses and physicians. Many doctors are arrogant, but so are a few nurses, so that isn't the source. The real source is that a small percentage of doctors are alcoholics, drug addicts, and/or dangerously incompetent. A larger percentage are sloppy or painfully behind the times. But except when subpoenaed to testify under oath in a malpractice trial, no nurse dares speak out about them, not even privately beyond other nurses who are aware of the facts. They would lose their jobs instantly.

They do their best to cover for such doctors, as does the hospital administration (which cannot afford to lose the business), but the long silence creates bitterness. In turn, nurses burn out more quickly than in other professions, which means higher turnover and higher training and orientation costs for new staff. Check the classified ads in virtually any large city newspaper. Observe the high percent of entries for nursing positions. Finally, if you really want to identify who the bad doctors are, run a survey of nurses on the physicians they would personally recommend. Then compare the compiled results with a list of the physicians in practice in the area.

On the other hand, nurses are not blameless. Some of them are equally incompetent, and a few escape from floor nursing by earning graduate degrees and progressing to administration. There they create new paperwork requirements for their underlings for whatever reasons. Floor nurses refer to them derisively as "the high heel club" in reference to their shedding of the uniform and easy hours.

Medical technology is another sore spot in economic terms— great for the patient but havoc on hospital planning. It's costly to acquire and even more costly to staff for it, even when it represents a new profit center. And as regards competition for patients, that problem must be considered in the context of excess capacity.

EFFECT OF EXCESS CAPACITY

The idea of excess bed capacity may sound like a winner, perhaps because it can be used in emergencies or as an untapped resource to provide additional health care. It doesn't work that way in practice. Excess beds are arguably the single most insidious cause of accelerating health care costs. The reasoning is not complex and starts with a brief history of bed capacity.

Before World War II, hospital costs were moderate. Ten dollars a day for a hospital room, with few additional charges, was par for the course. Physician and surgeon fees were equally modest. Sixty dollars for an appendectomy was on the high side. Perhaps this was because there were few policies to milk. The first insurance plan was initiated in 1929, but the next ten years witnessed the depression. Health insurance was not a top priority item. Less than ten percent of the population had policies. Whatever the case, the pricing kept these hospitals from excess building.

Things changed after the war. Insurance became popular, even though costs remained relatively low at first. But the returning veterans sired the "baby boom" and with it a demand for increased health care services. Naturally, new construction became the order of the day, fueled by the sudden burst of medical technology spawned in part by the millions of casualties incurred in the war.

Then, of course, the costs began to rise and in 1966 Medicare was enacted. That exacerbated the increases, and eventually the government was forced to apply the brakes. The most successful measure has been the DRG, limiting reimbursement to the type of case, not length of stay. This, plus the introduction of hospice programs for those with terminal conditions, reduced occupancy significantly.

Still, hospitals are reluctant to consolidate unused beds into "mothballed" wings. Part of the reason is psychological and part is because different types of patients are not easily mixed on the same floor, for example obstetrics, pediatrics, and neurosurgical. Each requires its own specialized nursing staff. So the empty beds remain distributed throughout hospitals and must be paid for. The floors remain staffed of necessity and the space heated, maintained and depreciated. But Medicare and some Blue Cross-Blue Shield agencies will not pay for it. Thus hospitals pass on these costs to commercial insurers, who in turn pass it on to individuals in the form of higher premiums and higher deductibles. They are in the business of making money, not reforming health care.

The consequence is that the costs continue to rise exponentially and thus in an attempt to abate this, hospitals compete for more patients and begin to fudge the medical records by inflating the seriousness of the condition or at least going out of the way to document every possible incident and condition of every patient in hopes of doing so. In a few cases, it has been alleged that some proprietary psychiatric hospitals have retain juvenile patients against the will of both the parents and the child.[5]

This raises the question: how much could be saved if all of the excess beds were shut down. An even more interesting question is: who would decide and by what authority. The answer to the first could only be determined by operation of a model for one or two years using actual data. Chapter 13 in this book outlines a way of doing this. As for the authority to order the shutdown of excess beds, that could only be done by law. It would be draconian, but the trade-off is that under full utilization of the remaining capacity, hospitals could be reimbursed on a per-diem basis rather than per case, adjusted for both the average severity of medical conditions and regional cost factors. More on this in chapter 6.

One last point here. Much has been made of the operating differences between profit and non-profit hospitals. The former are often held to be the primary reason for the excess costs. The reasoning is that they minimize free care by leaving it on the non-profits, sometimes by simply eliminating emergency rooms. There is some truth to this, but they also pay taxes while the non-profits disguise their untaxed earnings under the name *surplus*.[6] In short, this appears to be a red herring, although under a universal insurance plan with per-diem reimbursement, the rationale for remaining proprietary could be weakened.

EFFECT OF PHYSICIAN REIMBURSEMENT

The three sources of physician reimbursement are: (a) insurance, (b) direct payments from patients, and (c) salaries, fees, grants, and whatever paid by various institutions. At teaching hospitals, especially those that are part of medical colleges, these sources become so intermingled that it is nearly impossible to sort them out. But for doctors in private or group practice, the third source does not play a major role and the other two are quite clear (except for health maintenance organizations with salaried physicians).

The effect of this reimbursement scheme parallels the wisdom of Willie Sutton. Human nature gravitates to where the money is, and doctors are no exception. They, like every other professional, may hold to high standards, but they won't turn down higher income, especially when it's perfectly legal. The issue is whether this laissez-faire attitude can be tolerated much longer. Probably not, and if the schedule is wisely chosen, it could improve the distribution of medical care. Consider the effects.

The first is the ongoing trend to medical specialization that is inherent in the exponentially growing body of medical knowledge. No one individual can possibly hope to master all the fields. This doesn't obviate the need for family physicians, which used to be called general practitioners, but the criteria are broader and more demanding today. The problem, then, is not in specialization, per se, but in the proportionality between family physicians and the specialists.

That it is disproportionate stems from two reasons. Until recently, medical schools emphasized the technical practice of medicine, not the human side. The logic was that humanism is fine but it doesn't help much on the operating table. Then there is the matter of reimbursement. Surgical skills are held in higher esteem than counselling or diagnosis in internal medicine and hence are paid more per unit of time. Fortunately, the new emphasis in medical colleges on family practice, and the realignment of Medicare reimbursement formulas for physician fees, is reversing this.

The second is the ability of physicians to charge above covered limits. This has served as a deterrent to individuals seeking help and also "deterred" doctors from working in regions where they know they can seldom collect that extra income. The fault, however, is not entirely with greed. The paperwork and audits associated with reimbursement are frustrating at best.

Together, these two factors have worked against the equitable distribution and availability of health care, both financially and geographically. But if the fees were capped in a fair and just manner, and excess charges prohibited (indirectly by not reimbursing hospitals who practiced with any doctor who did so), then the problem would abate. Further, if the fees were set high enough, and the paperwork lessened, few doctors would have reason to complain. That would leave only the continuing potential for fraud. Chapter 12 outlines a few provisions on that matter.

EFFECT OF INDIVIDUAL COPAYMENT

The relationship between sources of funding and health care costs is not static. Who pays, and how much they pay, and when they pay, no matter how efficient the system may be, will exert a major influence on the total health care bill. This is part of the "free lunch" syndrome. If an individual thinks that someone else is paying the bill for services, they will tend to use more of them than if they have to pay for part of it on the spot.

It goes further than this. If the copayment is in the form of a reduction in pay, the motivation would be at a lower level because the copayment would be history. If it were in the form of an annual deductible, the motivation would be higher because of the high payment that would have to be met out of take-home pay before any services were obtained "free." But if it were in the form of a per-service or per-patient-day charge, then the motivational level would be somewhere between those two levels. The out-of-pocket expenses would be more gradual and in proportion to immediate benefits received. Figure 5-1 outlines the comparative advantages and disadvantages.

	Advantages	Disadvantages
Annual Premium	• Provides the majority of required funding • Makes employees and retirees sharply aware of the total cost of health care.	• To the extent that copayments are reduced, it can become too great a burden for low-income consumer units.
Per Service of per Hospital-Day	• Effective deterrent against overuse. • More equitable than annual deductibles. • Simplifies subsidization payments.	• Requires more paperwork, especially with respect to subsidized patients. • Will generate a lot of grousing.
Annual Deductible	• This is the most common approach at the present time. • A major disincentive against excessive utilization.	• Complex administration. Records must be kept on every individual and frequently transferred between states.

Figure 5-1. Forms of Copayment

The remaining form of copayment is indirect and would consist of special taxes on alcohol, tobacco products, and even junk food (which arguably contributes to obesity and malnutrition out of proportion to other foods). The first two products are already taxed, but the funds are not earmarked for health care and they are not severe enough to serve as a deterrent or as the price to pay for indulging in habits that contribute heavily and unnecessarily to the health care bill. On the other hand, a number of foreign countries do practice this, especially Canada with respect to cigarettes. And the state of Maine has placed a tax on junk food (technically a *snack food*).

One last point. Copayments need not rely on a single option. Inevitably, each covered employee and retired Medicare recipient would be required to foot part of the premium, which (as at present) can be subsidized for the indigent. They could also be required to pay some sort of up-front copayment, as indeed most insurance plans now require. The keys, then, are effective proportionality between premium contribution and up-front payments, and then within the latter, if it should be by annual deductible or per-service. The former is simpler and more equitable, and it can be pegged to generate the same revenue.

6

STRAWMAN

Concentration is the secret of strength in politics, in war, in trade, in short in the management of all human affairs.
-Ralph W. Emerson

Given: (a) the factors discussed in chapter 2, (b) the economic realities that protrude into ethical considerations, and (c) the respective centers of gravity for ethics and economics developed in chapters 4 and 5, the practical approaches to an effective national system are limited. In terms of funding, there are only two options. The first would expand Medicare in some form to cover all individuals. The second would standardize and mandate universal commercial insurance for all individuals not covered by Medicare.

But neither plan addresses the underlying problems in the existing system. They would only fuel them by pouring more money in, or alternatively, they would apply various strictures piecemeal that could do as much harm as good, except in the special case of putting a lid on fraudulent claims. Still, bear in mind one point: some systems are neither systematic nor capable of being reduced to machinery. That is especially true of health care providers. It is not true when it comes to streamlining the funding apparatus.

In short, the ideal would be to streamline the funding and then use that as leverage for reform as necessary without intrusion or micromanagement of the actual provision of health care services. The strawman outlined in this chapter aims at that configuration, which after discussion of related issues in chapters 7 through 11, resurfaces in more detail in chapters 12 and 13.

MODEL

The first chapter in this book previewed four aspects of systems theory: (a) the power curve, (b) centers of gravity, (c) interior lines, and (d) the law of averages. Subsequent chapters may have exhausted the patience of readers on centers of gravity, but the other three were given short shrift. The reason was that if the centers are clearly identified, the lines emanating from or to them can be redrawn to effect necessary change. That simplicity lets the system rely more heavily on the law of averages and less on administration of detail. In turn, it can ride the power curve and let managers and the courts deal with the remaining problems piecemeal.

The simplest way to do this is shown in figure 6-1. All funds except up-front copayments paid by individuals directly to providers, would be deposited into a single national account. These funds would then be distributed monthly to state insurance agencies. They in turn would reimburse hospitals and salaried physicians on a per-diem basis, and fee-for-service physicians and other outpatient programs on a per-service basis. Both forms of reimbursement would be indexed to prevailing regional wage structures, and the per-diem reimbursement would also be indexed to average severity of patient loads plus a supplement for residencies. Providers would not be permitted to levy additional charges for covered services, but would be allowed to charge what the market would bear for other services, especially cosmetic surgery. And coupled with this would be absolute control over the number and types of hospital beds and hospitals permitted to remain open.

Premium-type copayments would be collected by employers and the Social Security Administration (as at present). Up-front copayments would be borne by each individual or family. Annual deductibles would not be required, but the first-day of each hospitalization would carry a steep copayment; subsequent days, a significant one. Prescriptions would be pegged at 50 percent self-pay.

Low-income recipients and indigents would be subsidized by a variation on the existing Medicaid program to the degree that they were truly unable to pay. This could be implemented by ranges and renewed every six months with a photo identification card. Holders of these cards would present them to providers who would then bill the state agency for the unpaid recipient share. In this sense Medicaid would become merely a funding adjunct to the national system.

For covered items, there would be no limits, but of course the copayments might begin to mount. Those who could not afford them could apply for temporary relief under a revised Medicaid subsystem, and for others, the existing deduction permitted for Federal (and most state) income taxes would indirectly subsidize the cost. Alternatively, they could purchase a supplemental coverage policy from a private insurer, which is quite common at the present time with respect to Medicare (and CHAMPUS).

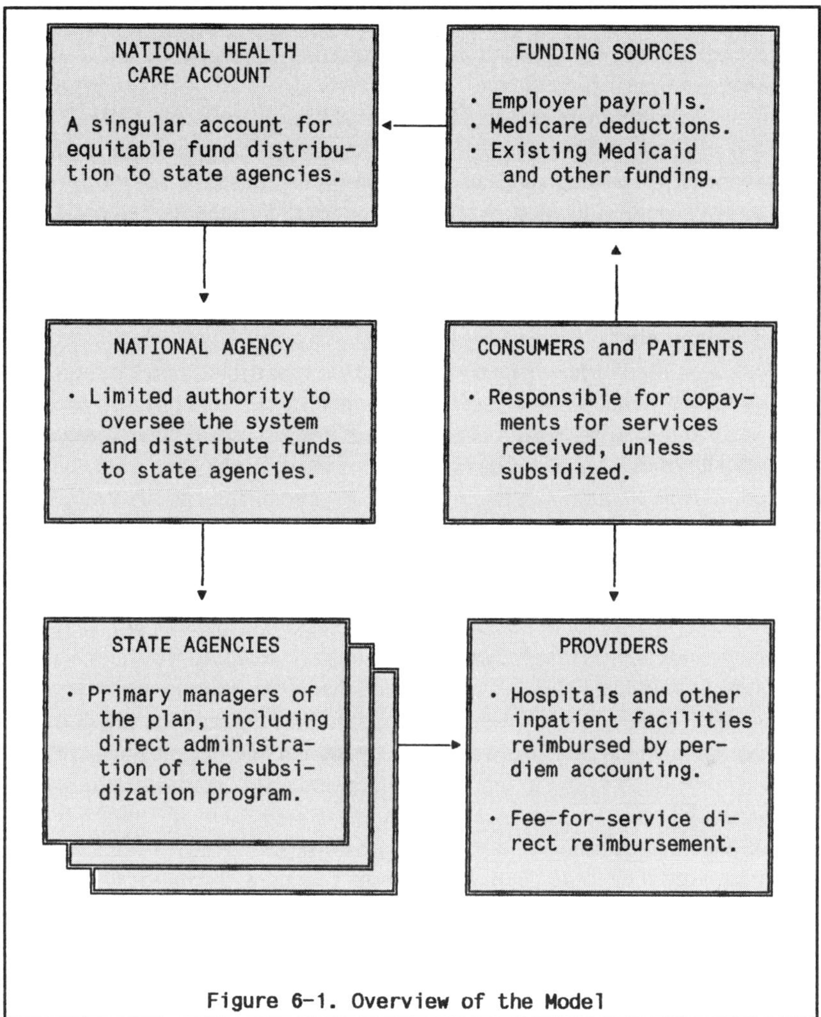

Figure 6-1. Overview of the Model

FACTORS AND ISSUES

For the interim, decisions on the scope and extent of coverage are less troublesome than they would appear, at least with respect to the model. Virtually all hospitals and all physicians would be covered, per se, but not necessarily for all procedures and services. For physicians, items not covered would not be reimbursed. For hospitals, the per-diem-based reimbursement would be reduced in proportion to the patient-days attributable to non-covered stays. For other providers, however, some hard questions need to be asked.

The second item concerns the source of revenue or premiums. Again, luck is riding with the model. Irrespective if the bulk of those premiums come from an expanded Medicare program or from a combination of Medicare and a tax on employers (and the self employed), the proceeds would all pour into the same account. The choice, therefore, would be immaterial to providers. The difficult questions concern the amount and proportionality of copayments, and the criteria by which individuals and families would be deemed to be low income and the extent of any subsidization. A related issue centers on the present option of Medicare recipients to waive what is known as Part B. This covers physician not hospital costs. If there is universal coverage, should this option be extended to all, or the opposite, removed from Medicare? If employees don't have the option, why should retirees?

And now for the $64 billion dollar question, and that's $64 billion per month. Precisely what services would be covered? This book makes no attempt to answer that question directly, but the developmental model for implementation outlined in chapter 13 would let the existing infrastructure address that question head-on over a two-year period. Will psychoanalysis be covered? If so, would it depend on the severity of the underlying problems? Would the copayments vary?

One last general point. If a national plan is enacted, the justification for many existing agencies and subsidies would diminish if not evaporate. All of the funds now poured into those programs should be diverted into the national plan if costs are to be contained. It's a wide net and there are a lot of unusual and rare species of fish in the water that most assuredly would be endangered. Hopefully, in this one case, they would be hounded into extinction. Moving on, then, to other concerns, the issue of how to fund government-owned hospitals would be the most pressing.

Of these, public hospitals and clinics are the easiest to deal with. They are usually supported by local, county, or state tax revenues, but under a universal health insurance, that would no longer be necessary, per se, although the system could continue to tax those jurisdictions for an equivalent amount. Veterans Administration hospitals almost follow suit. Again, if there were universal health insurance, there would be no need of a separate funding mechanism for these hospitals. Moreover, the majority of patients in these hospitals are suffering from non-service connected problems and could be treated in any hospital. True, the VA does perform additional services, such as certification or recertification for entitlement to veteran's compensation, but even that could be regarded and paid for as an explicit medical service. In short, the hospitals could continue to operate, and could do so under VA management, but it would be as if they were a chain of non-profit hospitals as far as funding is concerned.

Military hospitals, however, present a different problem. True, the vast majority of treatments at permanent station hospitals is little different than found in civilian counterparts, but troop unit hospitals, poised for overseas deployment, are a different matter, and much of the staffing in station hospitals is drawn from these units. The situation becomes more complex for retirees, who for the most part are covered under a special program called CHAMPUS (until age 65) but who can use military hospitals if space is available. Finally, personnel on active duty do not have copayments except for a minor charge for in-patient care as an offset against tax-free quarters and subsistence allowances already earned.

The ideal would be to fund station hospitals under the plan and cut the reimbursement to the extent the Department of Defense relies on direct funding of the equivalent of copayments, military physician salaries, and so forth, and then adjust that upon any deployment of personnel that are assigned to troop unit hospitals and the like. Thus it would not be necessary to integrate these hospitals into the civil sector—military training requirements would argue against it—but the funding could be streamlined and CHAMPUS eliminated, or more accurately it could be rolled up into the national plan.[1]

Another difficult issue would be reimbursement for health services obtained overseas, and this might depend if the individual were merely traveling, or working for a U.S. company, or working for a multinational, or for a foreign country, or just retired. At present and for the most part, Medicare offers no coverage here. Commercial policies, unless they are designed with that in mind, don't cover much here either. So it would not be unreasonable to leave health care coverage overseas to private or corporate supplementary policies.

And then there is the matter of funding support of medical education, and this depends on whether one is talking about a hospital that is part of a medical college, or one that has a residency program but is not associated with a college. The former trains students in medical school as well as residents. Teaching hospitals of both types tend to have a higher proportion of complex cases, but that would be taken care by a per diem rate indexed to the average severity of the patient load. The cost of training the students (who are sometimes called doctors orally but are not yet licensed to practice per se) and the residents is another matter. The model presumes that residencies would be funded; without them, the quality of medical care would self destruct. Funding for student externs would have to come from another source.

7

ANCILLARIES

*We are none of us tolerant in what concerns us
deeply and entirely.*
- Samuel T. Coleridge

The emphasis in the book thus far has been on hospitals and physicians. The reasons were: (a) the majority of the health care dollar is spent there, and (b) with the exception of long-term nursing and custodial care, few individuals will encounter back-breaking expenses for ancillary services, which by some definitions include any service that contributes to the maintenance of health. Still, any national plan that ignores them would be naive.

First, the providers will likely demand equal coverage under any universal system. Second, their indiscriminate inclusion would likely bankrupt the system much faster than would happen under a more conservative plan of coverage. Hence each of these services must be considered on its own terms, and further most of them may be subdivided under two broad categories: (a) orthodox services, and (b) alternative medicine. The latter ranges from near-orthodox practices to quackery that masquerades under the "alternative" moniker.

However, four items rate separate discussion: dentistry, pharmaceuticals, long-term nursing home care, and mental health. Dentistry is almost totally separate from other health care services. Pharmaceuticals are the source of the most pervasive controversies and legal entanglements in medicine. Long-term nursing care will eventually equal hospitalization in total cost. And mental health is so complex a subject that it takes separate chapter just to highlight the main issues.

To continue, then, data on ancillary services is uncertain. The primary difficulty is the definition or criterion of what is to be included. Does long-term care include assisted living arrangements? Do pharmaceuticals include non-prescription (over-the counter) preparations? If not, can exceptions be made when a doctor "prescribes" them, that is, recommends their use to a patient. When eyeglasses are prescribed, should a reimbursable prescription include only the cost of the optics or the frames too. And if so, does that extended to designer frames?

There is no practical way to reach a consensus on the criteria but one point is certain. As listed among the factors in chapter 2, if the health care pot of gold is consolidated into a singular funding source by way of Congressional legislation, then every conceivable provider and perhaps some new ones will emerge from the woodwork demanding a piece of the action under the banner "improved life for all Americans as part of the democratic tradition."

TABLE 7.1 HEALTH CARE EXPENDITURES

Item	1989 Cost	Percent†
Hospitals	$232,800,000,000	43.9%
Physicians	117,600,000,000	22.2%
Dentistry	31,400,000,000	5.9%
Other Professional Services	27,000,000,000	5.1%
HomeHealthCare	5,400,000,000	1.0%
Drugs/Other Medical Non-Durables	44,600,000,000	8.4%
Vision Products/Medical Durables	13,500,000,000	2.5%
Nursing Home Care	47,900,000,000	9.0%
Other Services	10,500,000,000	2.0%
InsuranceOverhead	35,300,000,000	—
Government Public Health	17,500,000,000	—
Medical Research	11,000,000,000	—
Facilities Construction	9,600,000,000	—
Total	$604,100,000,000	100.0%

† Excluding insurance overhead, public health, research, and construction.

Source: U.S. Health Care Financing Administration, Health Care Financing Review, Winter 1990.

The present numbers of that pot are listed in table 7-1. Excluding insurance overhead, government health services, medical education, and facility construction, the ancillary services for 1989 came to 33.9 percent of the remaining total or slightly over one-third of the health care bill, higher if the excluded items are factored in. And if the history of Medicare is any indication, those numbers would double if not triple under a national plan.[1]

As for the included items, "other professional services" covers registered and practical nurses on private duty, visiting nurses, podiatrists, physical therapists, clinical psychologists, chiropractors, naturopaths, and Christian Science practitioners. Durable medical goods include hearing aids, orthopedic appliances, artificial limbs, crutches, and wheelchairs. Insurance overhead includes Medicare processing but not claims processing expenses that are part of hospital operations. Further, many caveats apply, for example, the data on drugs do not include non-prescription items.

Next, nursing home care includes only the high end of the spectrum of assisted-living arrangements. That spectrum ranges from retirement communities to certified nursing care facilities that under a few circumstances and for a limited number of days are reimbursable by Medicare. To no one's surprise, the majority of patients in these facilities are elderly and that percentage may increase.

ORTHODOX SERVICES

Orthodox services are those that are fully accepted by physicians as necessary partners and adjuncts to the restoration and maintenance of health. Some points experience frequent debate, but most of the time those issues address the proper dividing line between them. And in one case, osteopathy, the dividing line has long since all but disappeared.

Doctors of Osteopathy (DO) are physicians and constitute a steady four percent of all doctors. In at least one state—California—MDs and DOs share the same licensure, and in all other states they are considered equivalents. About the only obvious difference is that some osteopaths continue to practice some elements of what amounts to chiropractic medicine (they use the term manipulation).

The next closest practice is podiatry, which is often thought of as a branch of medicine. It encompasses the care and treatment of certain foot disorders. Its practitioners earn the degree of Doctor of Podiatric Medicine after four years of medical training, and they are licensed to perform certain types of surgery and prescribe applicable drugs. Until this century, it was known as chiropody and dates back to the year 1500 BC. In short, podiatric medicine would of necessity be included under any national plan.

The next item—optometry—is equally orthodox. Optometrists also go through extensive training and must be licensed to practice, but that training is not as extensive as medicine (or dentistry) and they cannot prescribe drugs or perform surgery of any type. For that, they must refer patients to an ophthalmologist, who by training can also perform any service that an optometrist can, and some do. However, many existing insurance plans do not cover optometry services, and while the cumulative costs per person are not large, the total cost for a national plan would be in the billions. In a tight budget, then, this service would be one of the first on the chopping block.

The next service covers nutritionists and dietitians apart from those employed by hospitals but including weight loss clinics and specialists. The problem here is the lack of, or at least inconsistencies in, licensing and what constitutes practice hence reimbursable fees. Moreover, some nutrition/weight control clinics are owned and operated by MDs, a few of which are enshrouded in hype, charge vast sums, and make fantastic claims that have never been verified by scientifically credible tests. The only way this situation can be rectified is to develop nutrition as a medical support specialty under proper supervision with defined licensing criteria and the scope of services that may be provided. That is, nutrition is a very important aspect of health, but the quacks must be kept out of the cupboard.

Addiction treatment centers are another popular item.† Some of them are wings within hospitals, others are related, and still others are independent. They often advertise heavily and in some cases make high profits. The problem with inclusion in a national plan, therefore, would to avoid subsidizing excessive profits and to question just how many times one individual could use the benefits.

This leaves the original ancillaries: laboratories and radiology, although the technology has grown to the point where there are many new procedures, for example CAT scans. Although virtually every hospital has its own laboratory and radiology departments, many labs operate independently and provide services to individuals (or specimens, swabs, and samples provided therefrom) primarily on an outpatient basis as ordered by a physician. Hence, not much argument can be marshaled against including these services, per se.

The problem rests with physician ownership of some of them. Various studies have indicated that doctors who own these labs prescribe their services at a rate up to four times higher than doctors who do not have those financial ties.[2] Clearly, then, the only practical solution is to bar ownership or controlling financial interests in such labs by physicians unless that ownership is their primary occupation and they do not otherwise engage in medical practice beyond random emergencies.

DENTISTRY

If there is any group of providers that deserves special consideration, it would be dentists. At least four reasons apply: (a) they train as long and as hard as physicians, (b) with few exceptions they earn much less money, (c) they seldom win the gratitude of patients, and (d) the profession is being subjected to degradation by way of high-profit (for insurance companies) capitation plans. There's not much that can be done about the first three. A more solidly engineered national dental insurance plan could remedy the fourth.

These capitation plans are vaguely analogous to health maintenance organizations, where for a fixed fee per year (paid either by individuals or by

---

† One of the most effective addiction "treatment" programs is Alcoholics Anonymous, the original twelve-step support group. But because it is self-supporting and no person has ever been turned away because of low or no income, there is no need to include them in a national plan.

employers as a benefit), a wide range of dental services are provided as needed. Most of these plans have moderate copayments for prophylactic services and much steeper ones for restorative care. The problem with them is that they are based on the tendency of most people to avoid dentists unless it is absolutely necessary. This means that the policies are relatively inexpensive, and in turn the carriers contract with dentists to assume responsibility for a specified number of patients in return for a fix payment per patient per month, i.e., per capita, hence the term *capitation*.

For individuals just emerging from the high costs and debts of finishing dental school, there is sometimes no other way to begin practice. But the mechanics of these insurance plans encourage and sometimes force dentists to cut corners, especially if the assigned group of patients bucks the trend and visit their dentist more frequently.

The question, then, is whether to include dentistry in a national health care plan. Many arguments can be put forth for both sides of the issue, but three factors stand out: (a) as people grow older, and their funds begin to run out, they become strong advocates for adding it to Medicare (hence automatically to any national health plan), (b) dentistry is a self-standing profession and would only make management of the primary plan administratively complex, and (c) with rare exception, the cost of dentistry is infinitely more affordable than medical hospitalization. So except for dental care incidental to a medical injury, it would seem that any needed coverage could be better handled by an entirely separate plan and organization. And that plan will not come about unless the profession of dentistry takes the initiative to do so.

ALTERNATIVE MEDICINE

In previous centuries, the concept of alternative medicine had a strong impetus and justification. The practice of orthodox medicine was riddled with useless and even dangerous theory. Hospitals were unsanitary to the point where they probably generated as much disease as they served to cure. Effective drugs were few in number, and medical education was for the most part a sham. When the Flexner Report, criticizing medical colleges in the United States, was published in 1910, conditions had sunk so low that reform began immediately. The consequence was that alternative medicine, no matter how unsound it might have been, had about the same chance of success as the orthodox practitioners.

That just isn't true anymore. For example, naturopathy (not to be confused with neurology or neuropathy) is based on the theory that medical dysfunctions arise from accumulations of waste products and toxins in an organism and that symptoms are the consequence of the attempt of that organism to rid itself of them.[3] Treatments are centered on avoidance on so-called unnatural substances or "bad" environments.

Now it is obvious that toxins can kill and that "bad" environments can lead to terribly serious medical problems if not death. One only need consider the effect of eating certain species of mushrooms or ingesting chips of lead-based paint or asbestos fibers. And it is equally obvious that such behavior is to be avoided. But is that medical treatment? And will such avoidance eliminate cancer, coronary dysfunctions, stroke and diabetes?

Eliminate, no. Reduce the incidence of, probably yes, but it doesn't take a separate medical science to deal with it. The fields of nutrition and environmental medicine are perfectly adequate for the task. Therefore the need is not so much to shoehorn naturopathy into a national health care plan, as it is to further educate students in medical school on these aspects of medicine and to concentrate on elevating nutrition to a recognized support specialty.

Other alternative medical practices include homeopathy, acupuncture, chiropractic, and Christian Science. The latter is not especially Christian, as it often leads to death by ignoring the body of scientific knowledge, and by definition thereof is not particularly scientific. And in the case of children, courts have routinely overruled parents when the latter attempted to substitute a Christian Science practitioner for orthodox medicine. If, in such a case, the parents still refuse and the child dies, they can be, and usually are, charged with homicide.

Acupuncture is a different story because the benefits from some applications have been verified, replicated, and explained in pure medical terms. In these situations, then, it is being used as an adjunct therapy not as an alternative form of medicine. To some extent, the same is true of chiropractic "medicine." As an alternative form of medicine, per se, it belongs with the pyramids. As an adjunct treatment, say as occasionally practiced by osteopaths, it can be beneficial. A recent description by the columnist Peter Gott, MD, put the matter in clear perspective in a few paragraphs.[4]

And as for homeopathy (and herbalists), to the extent that its non-prescription "medicines" are effective is the extent to which it is orthodox and could be encompassed by a medical support specialty for nutrition. To the extent it makes claims beyond this, it is nonsense. In short, there is only one science, and that science demands rigid standards of testing and verification. except perhaps when experimental drugs and procedures are used in a last ditch attempt to save a life that would otherwise be doomed.

Unfortunately, science and democracy don't always mix. Science is based on facts; democracy on votes and emotions. Hence there's a good chance that every alternative practitioner will find his way in to any national health care plan unless the orthodox practitioners make a point of recognizing those specific practices that work as acceptable and clearly demonstrating the quackery of the balance.

For example, the *Encyclopedia of Medicine,* published by the American Medical Association, states: "Physicians believe that no scientific basis for chiropractic theory has ever been established ... "[5] However, with respect to osteopathic medicine, the same book states: "the osteopathic physician uses manipulation techniques, as well as traditional diagnostic and therapeutic procedures, to diagnose and treat dysfunction. Manipulation includes thrusting techniques and rhythmic stretching and pressure to restore motion to the joints."[6] Clearly, the two statements are inconsistent. It's a matter of giving credit where credit is due, and then nailing the rest.

PHARMACEUTICALS AND IMPLANTS

Take this simple test. Which of the two statements is correct:

a. Pharmaceuticals, which include vaccines and other inoculations, have been the single most important contribution in the saving and prolonging of life, and in the reduction of pain and misery, in the history of medicine.

b. Pharmaceuticals are the economic parasite of medicine.

Answer: both statements are probably correct. Paradoxical? Not at all. Whenever anything works well, enterprising corporations are sure to find ways of reaping more profits from it regardless of any lack of new benefits. And so no aspect of medicine catches as much flak as the pharmaceutical and implant trade. However, the insatiable appetite of many consumers for prescriptions, especially tranquilizers, doesn't help matters.

There's no shortage of literature on the subject, and the criminal negligence associated with silicon breast implants has of late been front page news. A recent two-part article in *Consumers Reports* outlined and documented much of the abuse in this field.[7] The worst of the abuses can be summarized as follows:

• *Lack of Effectiveness.* Of the more than 5,500 FDA approved prescription and over-the-counter preparations, perhaps no more than 10 to 20 percent have been proven to have any significant effectiveness *over and above what is already on the market,* at least for the 20 or so new drugs approved each year. This doesn't mean that newly approved drugs lack effectiveness, only that the effectiveness duplicates what is already available.

• *Promotional Hype and Biased Sponsorship.* Promoting these products has become a way of life for the manufacturers and has now extended to general magazines with endorsements from celebrities, who have not an iota of medical training, touting the advantages of certain pharmaceuticals. Worse, many if not most manufacturers sponsor supposedly objective seminars on drugs that in reality are thinly disguised advertising campaigns. This includes unjustified disparagement of generic, less expensive formulations.

• *Suppressed Negative Research Findings*. This may not be as common as the press sometimes suggests, but it is criminal conduct of the worst kind and in the most flagrant cases means pain and suffering for tens of thousands of consumers, witness the breast implants mentioned above.

However, there is one circumstance where chemically useless drugs nevertheless have therapeutic effect, and that is the placebo. Since time immemorial, doctors have known that some medical problems clear up or at least the symptoms abate because the patient believes in the efficacy of a drug that in reality is the equivalent of a sugar pill. This is no longer theory either; there is ample research to back it up, at least for some maladies. So allowance must be made for a few prescription placebo drugs, or alternatively, placebo counterparts to active drugs.

Whether the government will see its way clear to reforming the pharmaceutical trade is problematic, but there are a few simple steps that any national health care plan could employ to curtail if not eliminate the worst of the abuses. First, the plan could refuse to reimburse payment for any prescription that wasn't certified by the FDA as *being newly effective* compared to drugs already in the general formulary.

Second, all prescriptions for which reimbursement was obtainable would have to list both the proprietary and the generic equivalent, and leave it to the patient to choose. However, because generic equivalents of some proprietary drugs are in fact less effective and/or induce significantly greater side effects, physicians should be encouraged to point out that research to patients.

Third, in the event any manufacturer was found guilty in federal court of culpable negligence for suppressing negative information or findings on the safety or effectiveness of any of its products, then reimbursement for all of its products would be denied for a period of two years.

LONG-TERM NURSING HOME CARE

Long-term nursing care is expensive. In 1989, the bill for it from Medicaid alone was $20 billion dollars, and that just covers the truly indigent.[8] The reason, of course, is that the population is aging. That is, the percentage of people living past 75 years of age is increasing. This generates an increasing demand—swelling would be a more accurate term—for this type of care, one that will undoubtedly mushroom further if the government starts to finance it for everybody. For at the present time, many potential patients are kept at home for lack of funds. Moreover, advancing medical technology will tend to keep some of them alive even longer, albeit in a semi-vegetative state. Further, many home-based care givers would welcome the chance to get rid of their responsibilities. Finally, a growing elderly population means a shrinking worker base, and it is the latter who pay the taxes to take care of the former.

Clearly, this is a major financial problem but the sheer magnitude of the bill means that any pay-as-you-go plan will fail. The only hope lies in a long-term investment program, in which the premiums must be collected for a long period of time and invested (in business rather than funding the federal debt) and paid out as needed. And even at that it would still require stiff copayments.

8

MENTAL HEALTH CARE

*Fortunately, analysis is not the only way to resolve inner
conflicts. Life itself still remains a very effective therapist.*
- Karen Horney, MD

There's not much poetry in an operating room; there can be to life. That, sometimes, is the conflict between so-called physical medicine and psychiatry. Unfortunately, under any national health plan, that conflict would have to be resolved. Of necessity, any plan must have uniform coverage. Uniform coverage means reaching a consensus on what to include. That task is difficult enough with physical medicine. With respect to psychiatry, it's a major undertaking.

The reason is threefold. First, there are major differences between physical medicine and psychiatry. Second, psychiatry offers a much broader range and depth of acceptable therapies and treatments for many if not most conditions, especially when the closely related fields in psychology are included. Third, taken to a logical extreme, the attainment of mental health could evolve into socialism, where the government not only ensures that mental health care is considered a right but exercises the power to coerce individuals to conform to what is considered "normal" behavior.

That may seem like an exaggeration, but the incredulous prosecution of an unmarried mother in Syracuse, New York (cited in chapter 4) for the most asinine reasons indicates that the exaggeration is one of degree not substance. To continue, then, this chapter examines the major differences between physical medicine and psychiatry-psychology and then reviews the significance.

DIFFERENCES

For the most part, the practice of medicine is short term and aims, if possible, at restoring the status quo. In this context, health is often described as the absence of illness. A healthy person need not consult with doctors except for preventive medicine and early detection of problems that may be without symptoms at the moment—another case of "if it ain't broke, don't fix it." By contrast, the practice of psychiatry and psychology are often immersed in long-term treatment, and agreement on what constitutes "mental health" is anything but a settled issue. Some schools of thought hold that what is supposedly normal behavior is inadequate at best; more pathetic than rewarding.[1]

Related to this is the question of causes. Most physical conditions have physical roots, notwithstanding psychosomatic contributions and aggravations. Cancer, coronaries, and diabetes, are not products of the mind. Nor are most accidents, especially when the victim is an innocent bystander. Sometimes, one's mental health may prevent physical problems from recurring, or more likely the process of recovery may go further and faster, but treatment of acute coronary conditions and diabetes are not the domain of psychiatry.

The reason is easy to discern. Most individuals are born healthy, and most of those that are not have specific, identifiable deficiencies. With reasonably good diet and living conditions, most of the healthy ones will continue in that state of health until they reach 45 years of age or older. Hospitalization is infrequent between the ages of 15 and 44, and much of that is accident or war related.[2] For immediate proof, examine any age-indexed individual health insurance premium schedule.

Mental health does not follow suit. It is the product of genetic endowment and a lifetime of experience and learning. The proportionality is the subject of intense debate and undoubtedly it varies among individuals, but few practitioners hold that babies are born with perfect mental health and that only negative experiences detract from it. On the contrary, the attainment of deep-seated satisfaction and equanimity in the conduct of life is difficult under the best of conditions. When an individual has struggled through a traumatic childhood. it is an uphill struggle, one that is often lost.

On another level, it may be said that physical health is driven by chemical balances and imbalances, by functional or partially dysfunctional nervous systems, and so forth. By contrast, mental health is driven by emotions, by perceptions and the subconscious, by the ability to clearly see or not see the relationships between inner drives and motivations versus outward events and experience, and by the affects, which range from the experience of love, equanimity, and cheerfulness to hate, anxiety, and indifference. Thus many therapies in psychiatry and psychology are based on a conscious retracing of roots, from childhood if necessary. By contrast, physical medicine prefers rooting out a problem as it exists, or at least controlling it. How it formed or when it formed is usually less important than identifying immediate causes. Even when it is essential to identify those physiological liabilities, the intent is usually to control relapses or recurrences.

Still another difference is the concept of "normality." That term rarely inspires much debate in physical medicine. It's a different story in mental health. True, it could be and sometimes is defined as the absence of psychotic or severe neurotic conditions, which thus accepts most neuroses and a host of other shortcomings as "normal." Still, the vast majority of mental health problems, as gauged by the number of patients and clients rather than costs, are not psychotic in nature. Moreover, the road to health often depends on the make-up of the individual. Is it grief over the loss of a loved one carried too far or too long? Is it chronic depression stemming from an inability to manifest one's bona fide interests and talents? Or is it excessive guilt over past mistakes (or a lack of sufficient guilt or remorse over intentional acts harmful to others)? In short, normality in mental health is an elusive term and hinges on many subjective factors.

To this must be added the much wider range of acceptable therapies and treatments in mental health compared to physical medicine. With many physical disorders, acceptable treatments adhere to a narrow path. True, in some cancers, surgery versus radiation versus chemotherapy are options. And the debate on how much surrounding tissue should be removed, especially in breast cancer, drones on endlessly. But when it comes to mental health, one only need read the various theories of Sigmund Freud, Carl Jung, Alfred Adler, Karl Menninger, Erich Fromm, Rollo May, Abraham Maslow, Jean Piaget, Erik Erikson, Kurt Lewin, Harry Stack Sullivan, and M. Scott Peck, among others, to grasp the range here and the apparent irreconcilability of the various schools of thought.

The obvious compromise is that different individuals, at different times in their lives, can benefit from different approaches. Still, some of the options involve low cost counselling and no-cost support. Others, like psychoanalysis, can take five or more years and cost $50,000 or more. Further, the conflict over appropriate therapies for those conditions that are obviously disabling is almost as livid. Some professionals stress drug therapy; others, the one-on-one therapeutic environment; still others, family involvement, group therapy and support groups. Franz Alexander and Sheldon Selesnick, in their landmark *The History of Psychiatry*, put the case this way:

> And the struggle still goes on to the present day. The role of the devil has now been taken over by brain chemistry. No longer a devil but a deus ex machina, a disturbed brain chemistry rather than a person's own life experiences, is responsible for mental illness. Whatever the cause of faulty brain chemistry may be, the new conviction is that the disturbed mind can now be cured by drugs and that the patient himself as a person no longer needs to try to understand the source of his troubles and master them by mental processes...[3]

Another key difference is that mental health increasingly depends on involvement of the family or loved ones as part of the therapy, whereas in physical medicine this is often seen as merely supportive. The reason is that those relationships may have exacerbated if not caused the condition. As a minimum, the support by friends and loved ones may be necessary to help the individual over the hump, so to speak, in the absence of will power (a concept that itself is hotly debated) to go it alone. By contrast, the onset of insulin-dependent diabetes mellitus is rarely a product of family life, though the patient obviously needs the support of his or her family and can certainly do without any ridicule.

Another obvious difference is that while medicine is dominated by MDs, the same is not true in the field of mental health. There are more psychologists than psychiatrists, and PhD psychologists, and not just MD psychiatrists, are now admitted to psychoanalytic training programs. Further, physical medicine depends on physical intervention, be it the quick way by surgery, radiation or some equivalent; or by drugs, diet or similar. Bedside manner is nice to have, but most short-term patients will trade it for absolute competence on the part of the physician, especially in cases of surgery.

In psychology, however, something akin to bedside manner is critical. It goes by many names, among them "the laying on of the psychical hands." An even greater number of theories try to explain the effect and how it should be utilized. Some posit that the respect and love (in the most mature sense of that word) an analyst demonstrates toward a patient can instill a genuine sense of self-respect as the basis for any further improvement, especially if that patient had been deprived of it in their childhood, and hence this is the real source or at least the primary source of healing.[4]

Then, too, consider the literature written on the subject. Books on physical medicine are seldom popular. About 20 years ago, Gustav Eckstein's *The Body Has a Head* was the main selection of the Book of the Month Club, and the Lewis Thomas anthologies of his own essays are popular too. But aside from various one-volume encyclopedias (e.g., AMA, Mayo Clinic, and Columbia University), there's not much on the layman's shelf. Not so in the field of psychiatry and psychology. Walk into any chain bookstore, and you will find at least a hundred titles. Even Freud's works still sell in the tens of thousands of copies annually. Moreover, while the ancient treatises on physical medicine are often a source of hindsight humor, the works of the Greek tragedians and Shakespeare seem to be as valid today as ever.

SIGNIFICANCE

This leads directly to the debate on the role of character versus disease, especially when it comes to addictions. The concept of character is based on personal responsibility for one's actions. The concept of disease, by contrast, implies factors which are beyond the individual's to control. For polemics, the former says: "These are the facts and the law. If you don't mend your ways, these are the consequences." The latter says: "You are not capable of dealing with your problem. We are obliged to intervene to the extent that you cannot, or at least until that point is reached when can cope largely on your own."

Now obviously, when an individual is psychotic and beyond rational judgment, somebody has to intervene, although just what specific therapies can be forced on a patient is open to debate. Remember insulin shock therapy and prefrontal lobotomies? At the other extreme, no credible professional will advocate massive intervention when a family has a passively neurotic squabble over whether to go the beach or the mountains for a vacation. It's the stuff in between where the potential trouble lies.

This conflict is sometimes brought to the forefront in the courtroom when a defendant pleads guilty by reason of insanity. John Hinckley, who attempted to kill President Reagan, was adjudged insane at the time of the crime, and is still confined at St. Elizabeth's hospital in Washington, D.C. By contrast, the same defense failed in the recent Jeffrey Dahmer case, and he was sentenced to 15 consecutive life terms.

Although the difference between incarceration in a penitentiary and a ward for the criminally insane may not seem much different in practice, that is superficial to the thesis here. If the insanity defense fails, and the crime is capital, the individual can be executed. But if the insanity defense holds, the individual is no longer a criminal. He is a patient who can be released whenever psychiatrists certify (often with the concurrence of the courts) that the condition has been "cured" or at least abated sufficiently to let him or her return to a life of freedom. Fortunately, the number of insanity-defense cases are small. Unfortunately, to the extent that the insanity defense exists at all is the extent to which the state, and hence caregivers under a national health care system, could assume responsibility and forcibly place an individual under their control.

In all of this welter, then, one must ask: what are the centers of gravity? Economically, they still reside with: (a) psychiatrists, (b) short-term hospitalization for acute episodes, and (c) long-term care of the chronically ill. That is where most of the money is spent and to which most of the dramatic cases gravitate. But arguably the ethical center of gravity is the debate on personal responsibility highlighted by the various schools of thought and therapies. Nudging those two centers closer together is no small task. Thus it is in this arena that the definition of health and health care, and hence what will be provided, runs the greatest danger of slipping into absolute socialism.

9

EMOTIONALLY-CHARGED ISSUES

A fool may ask more questions in an hour
than a wise man can answer in seven years.
                              - John Wray, 1670

The story is told about the woman in Minnesota who lived on a farm adjacent to the Canadian border. A new survey found that the house itself was actually on the other side, and accordingly the officials paid a call to inform her of the situation. She replied: "I don't want to live in Canada." They went on to explain it was only a formality and that she would notice the change only in her new address and who delivered the mail. To this she again railed: "I don't want to live in Canada." This went on for several rounds, each ending the same way. Finally, one of the officials deemed it wise to ask her just why she didn't want to live in Canada. She responded: "Oh I hear they have such terrible cold winters up there."

Some issues bear less significance to the overall scheme of things than the publicity surrounding them suggests, yet their political effect is not to be underestimated. History demonstrates that a single event can galvanize a nation after thousands of logical entreaties fail. Pearl Harbor comes easily to mind.

Health care is no exception to the pattern. The growing costs combined with increasing unaffordability for many Americans makes for political hay, but some of the items on the front page are not especially germane to that scenario. This chapter examines several of them, concluding that any attempt by the system itself to resolve them would be akin to eating parasites to assuage hunger.

HIGH-COST PROCEDURES AND CATASTROPHIC EXPENSES

High-cost procedures are by definition catastrophic expenses except with respect to wealthy patients. To a billionaire, a quarter of a million dollars is one or two days interest on savings. To the poor, it is 20 or more years of toil. The same is true of high cumulative medical expenses. That variation may not be as dramatic as a heart-lung transplant, but the financial consequences are essentially identical after a year or so of accumulation.

In Bill Moyers' interview with Willard Gaylin, a bioethicist, the latter related that he once asked a physician how a liver transplant costing $200,000 was paid for. Without hesitation, the doctor replied "up front."[1] The significance of this is that for the majority of people, these expensive life saving procedures are beyond reach even with adequate health insurance coverage. But, so goes the reasoning, a national health care plan would correct that deficiency and open the door to all in need.

Yet the concern is raised that open door policies would incur unacceptable costs and therefore some procedures must be excluded or left to charity. Then sayeth the poor: "Health care is a right, but apparently it is a right that must be purchased. Only the wealthy can afford it." And as the costs go largely to cover expenses, even charitable providers respond that until the system changes this situation will continue, and thus support catastrophic coverage. Less charitable providers chime in too, but their hands are on their wallets not the hymnals. If this weren't so, why is the annual bill for fraud in health care now estimated to exceed $50,000,000,000?

To this, some critics respond that it is entirely possible to make all of this expensive care available at public expense, but ask if it would be good stewardship to invest those kind of funds in individuals who may have only a few years to live? With limited resources, wouldn't it be better to spend those funds where they could do more good for more people? Then they point out a practical problem. The short history of Medicare catastrophic insurance suggests that the option is not politically popular. That tax was graduated and levied primarily on the wealthiest retirees. They balked and got Congress to kill the plan the year it was implemented, implying that it should be paid for by the working class similar to other social security benefits, ignoring the fact that Medicare requires a premium and copayments and also imposes limits.

The real reason, of course, was that most wealthy retirees had already purchased supplementary Medicare policies from the private insurance market. As such they had little need for it and did not want to be taxed to pay the premiums for the less fortunate. This, incidentally, is in keeping with almost all of the surveys conducted by the American Association of Retired Persons, namely that the overwhelming percentage of retirees want reform and more coverage without paying additional taxes or premiums.[2]

Still, in all of this emotional welter, or perhaps because of it, the magnitude of the problem is exaggerated. It is true that catastrophic medical expenses may be financially devastating to a patient and his or her family, but only a very small fraction of the population will ever encounter this situation. Moreover, the total of all catastrophic costs for the entire country is only a small part of the $750,000,000,000 tab. For similar reasons, health insurance companies tout high limit major medical coverage of a million dollars or more but downplay annual deductibles and copayments of $2,500, or higher, per person per year. It is first dollar coverage that burns insurance carriers not the occasional big bill.

In short, the inclusion of catastrophic coverage in any health care plan would not be all that expensive, provided: (a) the potential for fraud were throttled, (b) copayment provisions were hefty without being destructive, and (c) the services were not showered on the terminally ill or on those for whom the procedures would do little to improve overall health.

That would still leave the issue simmering on the political back burner, and as Samuel Gompers once remarked when he was asked what the American worker wanted, his response consisted of one word: "More!" And so it will be with health care. Whatever is provided will never be enough in the long run. The beneficiaries will always want more, no matter what it costs, and the game plan almost inevitably will be "tax the rich." This potential situation, therefore, is the basis for including a brief discussion on distribution of income and taxes in appendix A. It may come as a surprise to some readers, but the poor pay almost no *net* taxes. On the contrary, tax credits for most low income individuals and families *with one or more children* results in a credit that more than offsets the FICA (Social Security) tax, while the wealthiest 20 percent of individuals and corporations still pay the lion's share of the taxes.

MEDICAL RESEARCH AND TECHNOLOGY

There are three types of research in all fields: (a) that which makes incremental improvements to known procedures and practices, (b) that which makes a quantum leap in the same direction, and (c) that which is truly revolutionary. An example of the first level would be a variation on the chemical composition of an existing drug that significantly increases its effectiveness, or, alternatively, makes it useful for a wider range of conditions. An example of the second level would by less intrusive laser or fiber-optics-based surgery that transforms a five-day inpatient procedure to a three-hour outpatient treatment. An example of the third level would be genetic manipulation during gestation that literally "re-formed" the errant genes that would otherwise trigger chronic disabilities. That last example may sound a little far fetched at the moment, but it's coming.

The dividing line between any two levels is not always precise nor do costs necessarily correspond with the level, but cost they do. So within the context of national health care, the questions are: (a) how should research and development be funded, (b) can the often piecemeal research be organized to make it more effective in the sense of time, and (c) should a greater sense of priorities be imposed. The last two are charged with emotion; the first is the really important one.

In the early 1970's, President Nixon decided to conduct "a war on cancer." All research was to be organized and prioritized in order to more effectively "conquer" this admittedly dread disease. But when the hoopla died down, so did the "war." The reason is that effective organization of effort is only possible when everybody knows what they are doing and understands the logic of the problem. This simply isn't the case when it comes to cancer; science has not progressed that far. Somewhat more may be known about the cause of coronaries, stroke and diabetes (the other three major killers) but the science of prevention and more effective treatments is still evolving. This doesn't mean that research scientists have become lackadaisical. Far from it, but nature seems reluctant to yield her deepest secrets, as it were.

The alternatives, then, are either to plow in more money or to limit funds to the more promising research and divert the balance to the provision of services. Unfortunately, plowing more money into the system may not offer any return on investment. The most dedicated and likely-to-succeed researchers are, for the most part, well funded. As for the opposite tack, one can always cut out or curtail the less promising research, but deciding on the criteria for the cut will prove difficult, and there is always the chance that an obscure, iconoclastic scientist ridiculed or ignored by his or her peers will find a priceless answer.

About the only compromise would be to emphasize funding for research in the seven or so categories of medical problems that account for 95 percent of deaths and debilitating conditions beyond than those stemming from accidents and the inevitable process of aging. But even there, the few suffering from less frequent dysfunctions and diseases will eventually demand equal time. Still, if a national health care plan is enacted, all funds will become much tighter. Priorities will have to be set and decisions made.

PREGNANCY-RELATED ISSUES

No topic in health care is more controversial than abortion. The debates on voluntary sterilization and artificial insemination seem to be limited to certain (primarily Catholic) hospitals and some individual providers, and can be solved by continuing to allow both to refuse to perform services of this type. Abortion is another matter and has fueled organized intimidation of both doctors who perform them and patients who elect it. Sometimes this intimidation extends to acts of terrorism.

One side of the argument posits that the unborn child is living and hence the aborting of a pregnancy is homicide. The only clear exception occurs when the abortion is a necessary side effect of a procedure to save the life of the mother, on the grounds that without it the child will be stillborn anyway and of course the mother will die. Saving one life is better than losing both. Additionally, many pro-lifers would make exceptions in the case of rape or incest. The motivation here must be compassion, because the logic is at odds with allegation of homicide.

The other side of the argument holds that a fetus, especially in the first trimester, is a biological extension of a singular organism protruding into its own uterus, of which the woman involved has the same right to remove as her appendix. True, so goes this position, the fetus will in most cases evolve into a separate living human being, but until that point arrives, or where birth could be induced and the baby survive, the choice remains with the mother to continue or not continue the pregnancy.

Unfortunately, there is no way to reconcile these polemics, Nor is there any way to scientifically prove which one is right or closer to the truth. Science holds that mind and body are one, conveniently overlooking death, when life "disappears" but the body remains. Pathologists are not charged with homicide when they perform an autopsy. So under this assumption, life would have to be present in the embryo even when it is only a single cell. But assumptions prove nothing; they can only be used as the foundation or axioms for theories. It is just as easy to argue that life occurs only when it is plainly in evidence, a phenomenon which obviously occurs at birth. Interestingly, that perspective is much closer to the scientific tenet of replicable, verifiable experimentation and evidence.

The consequences of this emotional conflict are both short-term and long-term. If abortion (except to save the life of the mother) is declared unconstitutional, then the issue in terms of a national health care system would be moot. The service would not be provided, although individuals would be free to travel to other countries where it is legal. The system only need care for the medical complications generated by illegal abortions, regardless if the patient is sent to jail or not. But if that right is upheld, then the system must provide and pay for it or elect to exclude it as a self-pay treatment along with, say, most cosmetic surgery.

That's the rub, of course. Any national health care system must respond to the electorate. The administration in power would find it a lot harder to impose or loosen controls by executive order. Still, no matter what the Supreme Court decides, or what political decisions are made, or perhaps what constitutional amendment is passed if it comes to that, the two sides will continue to fight it out. That will consume political capital that could be spent on more pervasive problems and issues in health care.

EUTHANASIA-RELATED ISSUES

The concept of euthanasia is even more laden with ethical difficulties than abortion. The reason, of course, is that by definition the conflict always applies to an individual who is living, not one that has the potential to live. Ideally, then, the resolution is simple. Euthanasia is homicide and cannot be tolerated. In practice, it's not that simple. The cases range from the decision of an individual with a terminal illness to forego extraordinary medical care and thus let nature take its course ("death with dignity") to the school of thought that claims once an individual becomes terminally ill or is afflicted with medical conditions that require permanent round-the-clock care, they have an obligation – a duty – to die and that the state should encourage them to do so and offer the means necessary to accomplish it. Almost everybody supports the first polemic, while the second conjures up images of Nazi Germany.

The complexity of this range intensifies when the individual is no longer capable of making such decisions, especially in comatose situations where there is no chance of recovery and the decision devolves upon a guardian. If the patient had expressed a preference (usually by way of a "living will") for terminating life under such conditions by having nutrients withheld, can providers or survivors overrule it? Support for living wills is growing, which is not true for Dr. Kavorkian's "death machine." As of this writing, he has again been charged with homicide.

Further, and unlike abortion, this issue does have major economic consequences. The bulk of health care costs are gravitating towards the elderly, and within that slice of the health care dollar, the amount spent in the last six to twelve months of life remains significant (28 percent of the care alone). As mentioned elsewhere, other countries have found it necessary to ration or otherwise limit care given to the elderly, especially those with terminal conditions notwithstanding the conflict with the medical ethic to preserve life.

OTHER ISSUES

Another emotional issue is the patient's right to refuse care except when it is court-ordered or the patient is a child and the law takes precedence over parental religiously inspired preferences to the contrary. In a democracy, no system can impose treatments in general, but if the refusal to accept care or follow medical advice in a timely manner leads to major but avoidable expenses later, should that individual be made to pay a larger share of the tariff? If so, what are the criteria and who will decide? How scientific are those criteria? Who will keep records?

Still another issue concerns provision of care for illegal aliens, and whether or not the country can afford to maintain current legal immigration and refugee policies. At one time the economic opportunities were so vast that we could absorb all comers. Today if too many of them remain on welfare, that might no longer be true. Consider also the acquired immune deficiency syndrome (AIDS) epidemic. Once manifested, the syndrome is always fatal, but it can take years to progress. Should the government foot the entire bill for every case (which goes far beyond direct medical treatment), and should so-called "aggressive therapy" be paid for in the hopes that a cure might be found within the slightly extended life span?

* * *

Ideally, the sound approach for health care providers under a national plan is to let decisions on these matters rest outside the system—to leave them to the political process and then respond accordingly. It won't work, of course, because providers themselves are also part of the debate and have emotions just like everyone else. Still, if coverage is mandated or conversely outlawed, there is little choice but to comply. All that can be done is to immediately assess the moral effect and financial cost with respect to existing providers and facilities. This was one of the primary reasons for outlining the automated analysis model in chapter 13.

To do anything more is to ask for trouble. The practice of medicine is still more of a hard science than a social science, more logical than emotional, more idealistic than political, notwithstanding extensive fraud and malpractice. Attempting to resolve political issues can only dilute that emphasis and would not likely lead to any satisfaction. An exception might be made for medical research, but as the pressure for wider coverage builds up without the money to pay for it, that research stands a better chance of continuing if it is separately funded.

10

AUTOMATION-BASED ISSUES

*Disproportion is the root of all moral mistakes.... Within most
virtues there lurks, waiting to slip its leash, a vice in the form of excess.*
- George Will

Automation was once regarded as an interesting management tool, good for
accounting and mathematics but too mechanical to be of much utility for other
professions. In the last fifteen years that image has changed drastically. Today
the country would probably come to a commercial standstill if every computer
suddenly went blank, and a good part of the work in health care would slow to
a crawl, especially the operation of laboratories and high-end diagnostic tools.

Still that isn't the problem. The problem is the intrusion and potential
misuse of computers in the management of human and professional affairs. This
potential is far greater than popularly believed. Automation offers many advantages and so the technology will likely permeate every aspect of health care
before the full extent of the side effects are recognized.

The advantages accrue in two related forms: (a) massing information into one
system or at least into integrated databases, and (b) the ability to draw sound logical
conclusions to support decisions in a matter of minutes at a negligible cost rather
than months and years for thousands of dollars worth of clerical labor. The side
effects include invasion of privacy, perniciously distorted information, and more
subtly, an overdependence on machine logic at the price of exercising judgment.

MASSED INFORMATION

Perhaps the best way to introduce this aspect of automated systems is to
highlight the experience with the National Practitioner Data Bank. This system
was mandated by Congress in 1986 with the intent of preventing doctors and
other individual providers from changing venue with impunity after they had
been nailed for malpractice and/or other inappropriate behavior in their former
locale. The four required inputs were and are: (1) insurance malpractice payouts,
(2) state medical board actions, (3) hospital actions affecting privileges, and (4)

adverse actions taken by professional societies. Among other users, hospitals must check this data bank for adverse information on all applications for appointments to their respective medical staffs, and every two years they must conduct a "checkup" on all current medical staff members.

Mechanically, the system works well, but its accuracy is often in question and the resulting damage to reputations has sometimes made the data bank guilty of malpractice in its own right.[1] Moreover, this "malpractice" stems from both inaccurate input and piggybacking additional functions and data on the system, a negative example of the power curve effect. Once an effective database is established, adding new data fields and records costs little but vastly increases the potential applications. And the abuse.

Still, the National Practitioner Data Bank is child's play compared to what computer science now has to offer. The first of those offerings is called *image processing*. Image processing can instantly record any document in any and all colors as an electronic image. If the system uses a network, that image can be retrieved on a computer terminal anywhere in the world in a matter of seconds. This could eventually include every medical record and notation made by every provider, thus increasing the amount of automated information available to managers by a factor of twenty to fifty.[2]

How long will it be before this becomes a reality? Yesterday. Virtually every major insurance company already uses it, along with Congress, courts, banks, manufacturers, legal firms, state and city governments, and several hundred others. The Internal Revenue Service is developing an image processing system that will eventually record every document submitted (except those that are already submitted in digital electronic form).[3] Investment in this technology exceeds a billion dollars a year and is rising fast.

The one technical disadvantage to image processing is that it consumes enormous amounts of memory and it takes more time to transmit an electronic image of a page than text that has been reduced to character-by-character data. This is because the image is recorded in hundreds of thousands of nearly microscopic dots (called *pixels*, for picture elements). However, that disadvantage is only temporary, and moreover while a user is reading the first page of an electronic "folder," the network can complete the balance of the transmission.

Of more significance is the development of fiber optic commercial trunk lines. The transmission capacity of these lines is so high and so fast that all of the existing and potential medical and health care related data in electronic form could be linked and become accessible to any user as if it were all stored on a single computer. This will make the systems foreseen in Aldous Huxley's *Brave New World* (and Woody Allen's comical variation *Sleeper*) seem Neanderthal by comparison.

For example, it is well known that two or more drugs, each prescribed by a physician without the knowledge of the other prescription, can be detrimental to the patient. This even applies to some combinations of prescriptions and over-the-counter remedies. So that problem could become the justification for integrating all medical records on every individual that any physician could check before writing a new prescription. And the logic behind this would extend to many other undeniably useful therapies that are dangerous only in combination or only with a few patients who might have an anaphylactic reaction or the equivalent. On an even higher level, complete records of this kind might lead to early detection of other problems by statistical analysis of comparative data.

That is not so far fetched. The Otis Elevator company can now accurately predict which of its elevators are about to break down, based on a continual, automated review of maintenance data.[4] With this, it sends out overhaul teams before the breakdown occurs, and that makes building managers happy. Health care is more complex, but with computer technology the capability is only a matter of time.

So far so good. But once a system of this magnitude is created, how could access be adequately controlled? Employers could bribe medical records clerks to access these records in order to identify psychiatric problems, former addictions, and other information that might work against being selected for employment. Keep in mind Thoreau's warning that "men become the tool of their tools."

PROFESSIONAL VERSUS COOKBOOK MEDICINE

The term "cookbook medicine" is the current moniker for what is more formally known as *prescribed protocols*. A prescribed protocol means that treatment of a specific condition must or should adhere to a set of standard operating procedures, complete with alternatives for most known variations that occur in practice. It doesn't bypass the skill of the physician but it does attempt to limit what should be done in the treatment of any disease or dysfunction.

Now there is a certain truth and utility to prescribed protocols, and they are inherent—in an informal way—throughout the profession of medicine. Else, medical students would never be able to put their learning into practice. The same is true for other professions including law and certified public accounting. To practice these professions requires the passing of examinations, and the questions and problems on those examinations bear all the hallmarks of prescribed protocols. So the problem rests not so much in the concept but in the excessive reliance placed on it.

In more detail, the expanded, formal use of prescribed protocols arose from the attempt to control costs and prevent unnecessary hospitalization by way of second opinions and peer review. Whenever these goals are implemented, there must be criteria, and those criteria are best developed by pragmatic review of thousands of similar cases—an application of the law of averages. And sure to form, most medical procedures do fit into patterns, but those patterns do not take into account the specific proficiency and experience of each doctor and therefore what procedures and techniques he or she is most competent with. Nor does it take into account the thousands of nuances common to most disorders.

The theory is that the law of averages will take care of the exceptions. For every treatment that takes longer or requires more expense, there will be one that requires less, a fact that has been derived from the averaging of thousands of cases. In practice, however, insurers and hospitals exert pressure on doctors to cut short the length of stay for complicated cases in order to improve revenues. And because all of this data has been reduced to automation, many doctors are confronted repeatedly with a printout of his or her record compared to others. Because these printouts do not always take into account the severity of the cases, it is easy to see how automation exacerbates the potential abuse.

DECISION SUPPORT SYSTEMS

Decision support systems combine automated data with programmed logic to mimic the human process of thought in order to support decision making. It theory, these systems are not a substitute for judgment, only a means of eliminating the tedious work of checking references, compiling and comparing masses of data, and presenting the "findings" in easy to read form. The danger is that the system will be perceived as the decision maker itself.

The history of these systems dates back at least to 1728 when Jonathan Swift wrote *Gulliver's Travels*. On his imaginary voyage to Balnibarbi, the character of Gulliver visits a university where the professors have created the first artificial intelligence machine. It consists of various words written on different faces of blocks that in turn are mounted on axles. The faculty cranks these axles at various speeds and then stops on command. Whatever words appear face up are scribed into a draft text and the process is repeated for the next sentence. Interestingly, Swift chose this for the only illustration in his book.

The intent, of course, was satire and while the machine he envisioned could have been built at the time it would have been of little use. It was based on pure random chance. One could do as well by playing darts with a dictionary as the target. The key word here is random. The idea behind decision support systems is to substitute logical progression for randomness. That step was taken in the 1830's. By then, Charles Babbage had invented the first mechanical computer, and Augusta Ada Lovelace (the only legitimate daughter of Lord Byron) developed the basis for programming it.

Her motive was not especially high-minded, for it seems she was prone to bet and lose fortunes at the race track and wanted a means of improving her odds by way of analyzing comparative data on the horses entered into any particular race. As Mr. Babbage never really finished any of his models, she never had the opportunity to try out her scheme. Still, her notes were not forgotten and her pioneering work was recognized in this century when the Department of Defense named their new programming language—Ada®—in her honor.

The concept of the decision support system lay dormant until the middle of this century, when it became known as artificial intelligence, and over the past twenty years, this endeavor has progressed from laboratory curiosity to practical application. With respect to the practice of medicine, the best known applications are in the field of medical diagnosis, for example the Mycin program. In a test of a variant on this, emergency room physicians were able to accurately diagnosis coronary conditions only 78 percent of the time using their judgment alone. With the support of the system, that accuracy rose to 97 percent.[5]

How these systems work may appear complex, but at core the development and processing is simple. Programmers and experts work closely together. The former writes down in detail the thinking (and data) used by the latter to arrive at a decision. The programmer then puts that into automated form. At juncture points where the expert must exercise judgment, the program pauses. For whenever a decision must be made, even to progress further in an analysis, that decision must choose from among options. That choice will likely be based on which option has the highest probability of being the correct one under the circumstances. If it leads to a dead end, then the next most probable path is followed. This is what is meant by an interactive system. True, there are no known programs that substitute for human intuition to "see" a brand new path to travel, but discoveries and inventions are rare compared to the sheer volume of day-to-day work done in any business.

In more specific terms, figure 10-1 depicts the range of applications in health care to which decision support systems can be applied, including the potential excesses. The breakdown is by the type of underlying logical structure rather than application, because the latter is too extensive for discussion here.

• *Actuarial Determinacy.* This is a more formal name for applying the law of averages to a mass of related data, of which the most extensive application in health care is the DRG system of hospital reimbursement for Medicare inpatients. Details on specific cases cannot be predicted with any accuracy, but averages of many similar cases operate almost as if they were adhering to laws of physics.

• *Linkage for Known Order.* The National Practitioner Data Bank is the archetypical example here. The existing data is known to fit a pattern but is too widely distributed to be of much use to higher level management. By consolidating it in one system, that problem is overcome.

• *Exceptions to Order.* This is related to the first two categories, but the emphasis is different. The idea is to highlight the outliers and then determine why. The IRS relies heavily on this technique to identify returns that are most likely in need of an audit. The program is called the Discriminant Function System. Within the practice of medicine, the technique has been used manually for thousands of years to aid in the diagnosis of disease.

• *Patterns in Apparent Disorder.* Integration or synthesis of scientific research has been the most fruitful application in the practice of medicine so far. This technique makes the forest visible in spite of the density of the trees, often by detecting trend lines, provided the trees—the research—are alive with accuracy. It is the most complex of the four categories.

	APPLICATIONS	EXCESSES
ACTUARIAL DETERMINACY	• DRG system of hospital reimbursement for Medicare patients • Potential for per-diem rather than per-case hospital reimbursement	• The high-enders are often pressured to reduce care and length of stay in order to increase overall revenues.
LINKAGE for KNOWN ORDER	• National Practitioner Data Bank, which holds information on actions reflecting negatively on the competence of licensed practitioners	• Erroneous data is easy to slip in. • Systems are easily expanded beyond the original intent and then abused.
EXCEPTIONS to ORDER	• Detection of fraud and malpractice by identification of unusual data within a mass of related data on peers and colleagues	• Bona fide variations can be erroneously faulted. The burden of proving otherwise then falls on the accused.
PATTERNS in APPARENT DISORDER	• Integration or synthesis of research data and findings • Analogous applications for health care management and financing	• It is easy to make loose assumptions and thus link data and findings that have less affinity in reality.

Figure 10-1. Types of Decision Support Systems

In summary, then, the critical task is not the equivalent of disarmament for automation. There's no stopping this technology. It makes too much money for the manufacturers and software publishers and the trend in management is to control everything in detail. Rather the task is to put a brake on misuse. There are several ways to accomplish this.

The first would be to limit access to data at the national and state levels of management, even if it takes Congressional legislation to effect this. Interestingly, a few corporations have backed away from micromanagement of field operations, including the Otis elevator case cited above. It reduced profits.

The second would be to dispense with or at least limit peer review and its accompanying automation to bona fide quality control under the primary supervision of providers (rather than auditors) and instead rely on closing down excess hospital capacity and a per-diem rather than per-case reimbursement formulas for hospitals. Fraud and malpractice can more easily be identified by reviewing overall claims at the state level with exception-to-order decision support systems.

The third is inherent in the first two, and that is to reinvigorate the sense of professionalism within the practice of medicine in lieu of increasing day-to-day controls. This does not mean abolishing the National Practitioner Data Bank, but it would mean restricting its use to the intended purpose and imposing severe penalties for intentional input of faulty data.

11

INFRASTRUCTURE

The functionaries of every government have propensities to command at will the liberty and property of their constituents.
                                                            - Thomas Jefferson

Infrastructure is often a polite word for inertia and the preservation of interests. With respect to health care infrastructure, *Newsweek* recently said that any reform proposal would have to gain the acceptance of the most powerful interest groups in the country, including hospitals, physicians, attorneys, labor unions, major corporations, insurance companies, and millions of retirees adamantly opposed to tax increases.[1] It should have added the government itself, because under Medicare and Medicaid the Department of Health and Human Services has become a major player.

Each player has vested interests in the present health care system, and although most of them advocate reform they do not want it to be at their expense. In theory, this would exclude increasing insurance coverage because that will raise the bill for someone. It also excludes limiting facilities or coverage, for that too will generate problems. And it excludes tightening controls, because that would visit more angst upon the providers. Perhaps the only hope lay with the battalion commander who during some intense fighting in World War II radioed back to his regiment: "They've got me surrounded again, those poor bastards!" More realistically, any reform of health care must have a balance of trade-offs, and those interests that will be cut the hardest must be seen by the majority as peripheral to the real needs of both providers and recipients.

RESISTANCE AND PRESSURE POINTS

Change in any form will always be resisted, and this resistance usually takes one of five forms:

• *Non-starters.* A non-starter is a plan that lacks sufficient horsepower to make it to a vote. The majority of proposals in all organizations, from households to Congress, probably fit into this category. This doesn't mean they won't resurface later, but the opposition recognizes the situation and lets the plan or proposal die a natural death rather than stir things up.

• *Skunk Farm.* When opponents believe that a proposal has a significant chance of being implemented but lack the necessary logic or clout to intercept it, they often turn it into a skunk farm. This means that by way of emotional overtures the plan or proposal is made to reek so badly that the deciders will decide it is untouchable. This approach, or at least attempts at it, is now par for the course in political campaigns and in confirmation hearings for Supreme Court justices. A common variation occurs when budget reductions are in the offering. The targeted organizations retaliate by threatening to close down one or more popular programs or sites. A few years back, even the benign National Park Service succumbed to the temptation and indicated it might have to shut down the Washington Monument if certain cuts were enforced.

• *Tunneling.* This approach is one of two taken when opponents accept the inevitability of reform, and then tunnel through the implementing rules so that they, and not the planners, control the purse strings. This is a common practice among corporations and others supposedly regulated by the government. The drive-up window at the Treasury Department is a myth only in the literal sense.

• *Zoning.* When tunneling is impractical, the alternative is to make exceptions for vested interests. Virtually every general tax bill that has ever been legislated exempts, at least temporarily, a substantial number of corporations and classes of individuals from the full bite of the provisions. Even the Constitution of the United States grandfathered the slave trade for 20 years and went so far as to prohibit any amendment to the contrary during that time.

• *Debate.* The debate approach means that advocates and opponents mutually recognize the validity of each other's arguments and attempt to resolve issues by open discussion. This is not uncommon in some town meetings and apparently was the key to the success of the Constitutional convention in 1787, notwithstanding the one instance of zoning. The approach is also common in appellate courts and remnants can still be found in education, but it seems to have recessed from the political arena.

At the moment, the proposal outlined in this book, or any reform plan, is a non-starter. The changes would be too drastic for too many parties, notwithstanding any built-in trade-offs. But costs keep accelerating and eventually payment for health care services will become a bona fide crisis. When that occurs, the ideal would be to aim for the debate level. That failing, and it probably would, the fallback is to the zoning level.

It was for this reason that the two-year study plan, as described in chapter 13, was prepared. It is important to ferret out the intransigent opponents while accommodating the bona fide needs of providers and consumers. Some of the opponents will eventually wash out but others will force compromise, read *zoning*. To continue, then, it would do well to consider the pressure points.

Opponents of reform usually oppose it for one of four reasons: (a) they will lose relative control or power, (b) they will be excluded to some degree, or what is the same, not be included in sufficient measure, (c) they will lose revenues, or (d) they will suffer a loss of prestige or professionalism. This applies to any kind of reform, from politics to theology to new theories in science. Failure to grasp the significance of these pressure points can only hurt efforts to attain objectives.

Understandably, parties that benefit on these fronts, especially if they gain on all four, will seldom be among the ranks of the opponents, but even when opponents are in the minority they have the advantage of being established. Successful reformists must either spark a revolution or persist in engineering the necessary horsepower to eventually prevail. As revolution is out of the question, a methodical approach to balancing these gains and losses is the only hope. Figure 11-1 on the following page outlines the potential gains and losses for the various elements of the health care infrastructure, which are then discussed in subsequent sections.

One last point before the specifics. All of the parties except unions (which don't need them) have one or more associations to plead their respective cases. Of them, perhaps the best known are the American Medical Association (AMA) and the American Association of Retired Persons (AARP). In years past, the AMA earned a reputation as reactionary and vigorously opposed almost every attempt at reform. But as many if not most doctors grew wealthy on Medicare billings, and the balance raised their fees in tandem much faster than the rate of inflation warranted, the resistance softened. The AMA may not have moved to the forefront of reform, but the change is significant and their most common complaint—that the government has intruded too far into the prerogatives of professional medicine—has some validity.

The other association—AARP—has in excess of 32,000,000 members, most of whom are drawing Social Security and are eligible for Medicare.[2] All but a handful of the balance are between 50 and 65 years of age (more older than younger) and so on average will become eligible for Social Security and Medicare in about five years. As such, AARP is the most powerful lobby in the world. Moreover,it is growing stronger and is the closest thing to a unified spokesman for the consumer, notwithstanding the more research-oriented *Consumers Union* (which often publishes major articles on health care for its sixteen million members). Finally, AARP has not limited its perspective to the elderly but clearly recognizes that the success of any reform must apply to people of all ages. Unfortunately, its current health care proposal (as reviewed in appendix D) advocates unlimited care of all types without sufficient controls. Moreover, the bulk of the new benefits would accrue to the elderly while the payments would fall almost exclusively to the working population.

	GAINS	LOSSES
Government	The obligation to ensure that health care is provided to all individuals at a reasonable cost would have been met.	It must stop micromanagement and second guessing professionals, fraud and flagrant malpractice excepted.
Hospitals	They would be free of claims processing and dealing with dozens of insurance carriers.	Thirty to forty percent of capacity would be shut down, including some entire hospitals.
Physicians	Payment in full from each patient would be virtually guaranteed, and billing would be vastly simplified.	No surcharges could be levied for covered services, and income of medical specialists would decline further.
Insurance Industry	Blue Cross-Blue Shield would likely become the dominant player, and spokesman for providers as well, under a much simplified system.	Except for long-term, overseas, and supplementary policies, few carriers would remain in the health care business.
Suppliers	Faster and more reliable payments from the hospitals that remained open.	With reduction of hospital capacity, total business would be down.
Business	The proposal would bring the continuous hassle on health care benefits to an end, except for supplementary coverage.	The total cost per employee would likely go up, primarily to cover subsidization of the indigent.
Unions	The long-standing goal for national health care would have been met.	Bargaining for supplementary coverage would be a tough road to hoe.
Consumers	The main problems of availability and affordability would have been solved, especially for catastrophic expenses.	Eventually, the cost per individual will rise and rationing in one or more forms will be imposed.
Attorneys	Malpractice suits would remain as lucrative as ever.	Jurists must confront the implications of health care as a right.

Figure 11-1. Political Battlelines

GOVERNMENT

The government is already the single largest and certainly the most influential player in the health care business. The resources include Medicare, Medicaid, CHAMPUS (the military dependents and retirees health plan), Veterans Administration hospitals, Department of Defense hospitals, the Public Health Service, the Food and Drug Administration, state, county, and city public hospitals and clinics, state licensing boards, the Federal Bureau of Investigation (which recently assigned fifty agents to help root out the estimated $50 billion dollar a year in health care fraud), and many others.

Additionally, it is Congress that has become the prime force behind a national health insurance plan, notwithstanding the opposition of the current administration to anything more strenuous than insurance premium subsidization. To this must be added the courts because they adjudicate malpractice suits and will be forced to dig themselves in much deeper if health care is declared a right. In fine, the government owns or operates perhaps a fourth of the pie and has its fingers in most of the rest.

The trade-off in this proposal would be to solve most of the major problems the government seeks to tackle in return for putting some distance between at least the federal level and the prerogatives of hospitals, physicians and other providers—a plan with teeth but not fangs. That means getting out of the micromanagement business. The one exception would be the prosecution of outright fraud (as clearly differentiated from malpractice). Felons yield only to ruthlessness.

NON-GOVERNMENT PROVIDERS

As developed throughout this book, non-government providers can be subdivided into in-patient facilities and fee-for service individual or group practitioners. Practitioners include physicians, podiatrists, dentists, optometrists, psychologists, and about 20 other classifications. The primary exception applies to those Health Maintenance Organizations (HMOs) that are hospitals combined with salaried doctors. (Other HMOs are largely local insurance plans that indemnify one or more hospitals and member physicians for specific services.)

Private hospitals can also be divided into profit versus non-profit categories, but there is little evidence the difference is a major factor except in the amount of "free" care rendered. And that difference would by eliminated by universal funding. The non-profits can also be subdivided into parochial versus non-sectarian, but this too has become a minor distinction except in the refusal of some of the latter to perform certain elective procedures related to pregnancy and sterilization. A third division would focus on teaching versus non-teaching hospitals, but except for those that are integral to a medical college, the effective difference is a somewhat higher mix of more difficult medical cases plus salaries for the relatively low paid residents.

Thus hospitals would present a more unified block of votes, so to speak, than might appear from their apparent differences. The one exception would be long-term nursing care and other custodial-type facilities. With the aging population, these have become high profit big business but often with a shady record for mistreating and abusing patients. Even some Catholic hospital systems have converted their nursing home facilities into profit centers. One in Tucson, Arizona, charges from $91 to $249 per day ($33,215 to $90,885 per year), plus supplies such as adult diapers.[3]

Hence there should be little doubt these long-term facilities will demand inclusion or that failing an equally generous federal subsidization, especially as some doctors have major financial interests in them. The proposal doesn't see it that way. Long-term care is a major financial problem, and according to *Consumer Reports*, the vast majority of available insurance policies aim at high profits rather than real benefits.[4] More importantly, the parameters differ too widely to package it with the mainstream of health care. It is primarily custodial, not medicine, and needs to be dealt with on its own terms.

For short-term acute-care hospitals, however, the most far-reaching negative would be the shutting down of between 30 and 40 percent of the existing beds. In practice, this means that a substantial number of hospitals would be closed. Of those that remain, the claims processing departments would be reduced to a shadow of their former selves. On the physician side, doctors would be obliged to accept payments from a regionally adjusted scale of fees (including patient copayments) without surcharges, at least for covered services. Moreover, those payments would be indexed to the amount of service rendered not to specialty skills (hence providing incentives to more equitably distribute the mix of family practitioners and specialties). Doctors would also lose influence over hospitals, as the funding would almost reverse the present situation.

On the positive side, the government would have to call off the auditor dogs and leave professionals to do what they have been trained to do, and to do it in their best judgment. Fraud would not be tolerated (nor necessary in the case of the hospital Robin Hood form), and malpractice would still lead to the courtroom. But the reimbursement would be set to continue the medical profession as the highest paid job classification in the country, and hospitals would gain the financial breathing room they need to operate.

Then, too, the old problem of providing free care would evaporate. Assuming subsidization of copayments for the indigent, every provider would be paid the same for the same service regardless of the economic status of the recipient. The danger, of course, is that once in place the federal government could garrote providers by cutting back on the reimbursement schedule. If a depression occurs there would be no other choice, but that would happen anyway under the current system. The way to prevent this is to establish payment thresholds that by law could be lowered only by an Act of Congress, not by administrative fiat, the same as is now true of Social Security benefits.

INSURANCE INDUSTRY

The health care insurance industry can be neatly divided into Blue Cross-Blue Shield agencies, which are all non profit, and the indemnity companies, which are mostly proprietary. In this proposal, the former would likely become dominant but streamlined, while most of the latter would be forced out of the arena, save for optional supplementary policies to indemnify individuals for copayments, and until additional reform is enacted, long-term care policies.

The reason is simple. The proposal would depend on state insurance (or more accurately state management and processing) agencies similar to the regional processing centers established for Medicare and CHAMPUS claims. Blue Cross-Blue Shield is already the dominant player here, and although proprietary insurers could (and should) compete for the contracts, the Blues will likely win out in most cases. They have the proven infrastructure and expertise.

Yet as mentioned, they would be streamlined. First, there would be no policy sales and management. Second, claims processing for hospitals (Blue Cross) would be reduced to per-diem accounting, which would be based on the average mix of DRG patients over the previous six months or so. Third, claims processing for fee-for-service providers would remain, but the payment schedule would be indexed and subject to negotiation only on the point of regional cost adjustments. The one added element would be to subsume the present state Medicaid departments to certify eligibility for subsidization of copayments. This would also entail direct payment of those subsidies to providers.

The subtle point to all of this is that Blue Cross-Blue Shield carriers are highly skilled at balancing the conflicting interests of the government and providers, and this skill would be essential to ward off intrusion on the part of the former. As such, they would become a primary spokesmen for providers, and beyond adhering to the general rules of the game established by Congress, they should side with the latter in bona fide conflicts. That is, the organizational set-up must make them independent of the federal government beyond narrowly defined controls. Those controls will keep the costs in line and ensure equal access, beyond which the government needs to retreat. This point isn't nego-tiable. Providers would not buy into the plan unless they were assured the dividing line was permanent beyond reasonable doubt.

SUPPLIERS

Suppliers range from linens to laboratories and pharmaceutical manufactur-ers, plus construction companies when it comes to building or modernizing facilities. The vast majority are proprietary and most of them would stand to lose some business if excess hospital capacity is shut down. And if more stringent measures are imposed on the use and reimbursement of pharmaceuticals and implants, the results would be similar to a formal bridge tournament held in Baltimore, Maryland some 15 years ago. Funds were tight that year, so the members had to share a facility with a dog show. Midway through the tournament, officials issued a bulletin lamenting the yelping and howling, adding in extenuation that the dogs were bearing with it very well.

What is there to say further on this? Suppliers are indispensable to the provision of health care, but they are dependent not independent players. The goods and services necessary for health care will be bought; those that are not necessary would not be bought. It's called the marketplace and the superintending economic philosophy is called capitalism.

BUSINESS AND UNIONS

At one time labor unions were the prime movers behind national health insurance, but that is no longer true. Perhaps the reason is that most of them have won ample health insurance benefits for their members, plans that may be even better than what a national plan would cover, especially in the way of lower deductibles. And business pays the bill in the way of benefits. Business also pays half the cost of the Medicare bill by way of the employer's share of the tax and collects the employee's equal share. So the unions should have few complaints if a national health care plan is established. If the copayments are higher and the coverage less than at present, they could always negotiate for supplementary policies.

As for corporate American, it knows that it must remain the primary collection point for funding health care. And whether that funding is called a tax or a premium is immaterial. What they want is equity and predictability, for example what share of the tax or premium would be paid by the company and what share by the individual. Because of tax consequences, that is a major point, but a flat tax *rate* applied to all earnings would be as consistent as possible with the current Medicare funding. Disincentives applied to consumers to deter abuse of the system are best handled by copayments, not additional payroll deductions.

CONSUMERS

The consumer will always be happy if he or she can get more care, under higher quality control standards, at less cost, closer by. This won't happen, at least not for all consumers. Rationing in some form will prove inevitable, even if all excess capacity is shut down and physician reimbursement is capped on a per-service basis. The federal debt is probably reaching the upper limits of the ability of the economy to finance it, not to mention what will happen when the government must begin to pay back the enormous debt it owes the Social Security fund.

But if the system is equitable, the indigent taken care of, the costs controlled, and the administrative costs frugal, then the remaining complaints would have little substance.

12

ORGANIZATION AND RESPONSIBILITIES

Experience is wonderful. It enables you to recognize
mistakes when you make them again.
Anonymous

Shortly after a resident of Boston retired to the southwest, a few neighbors began to rib him on the worsening standard of living in his native state. Sadly he admitted to some truth in the allegations, then added quickly: "But you know, Massachusetts was once a very good place to live. Up until 1620." Needless to say, the plan envisioned in this book would be a radical departure from the existing way of doing business and there's no guarantee its implementation would improve the resident system, or that the new infrastructure would be any less subject to the entanglements that mark the existing model.

The value of comparative infrastructures is for history to write, but one thing is certain: there would be a lot less of it. Still, the system that invokes organizational simplicity must also respond to the complexities of health care that no system can reduce. This chapter takes a first cut at that balancing act. It intentionally sets up an organization that will have to slug it out on many issues. When it comes to professional prerogatives, the weight is on the side of the providers. When it comes to the general operation of the funding mechanisms, keeping excess hospital capacity closed down, and prosecuting fraud, the weight shifts to the government. That is the nature of the beast, and any attempt to subvert those prerogatives in either direction could be fatal to the operation of any national health care plan.

STRUCTURE AT THE NATIONAL LEVEL

As presented in chapter 6, the organizational structure would have three levels: (a) the singular but limited national agency, (b) state-level (and equivalent) administrative agencies, and (c) providers. Figure 12-1, which is a variation on figure 6-1 (page 43), depicts it. The description here is as if the proposal were operating at full-scale and included all public and VA hospitals, at least from a funding standpoint. That may be a poor assumption, but it is easier to excise them during planning than to attempt to wedge them in later. It would also give those providers a better perspective on whether to buy into it.

The plan itself would initially cover most of the services now provided under Medicare and most Blue Cross-Blue Shield plans, notwithstanding that the agreement on specifics would take considerable analysis. It would not include payments for health care overseas; that would have to be covered by private insurance or other arrangements, which is the current rule in Medicare. The reason is that the system would have no control over those costs and billing procedures hence it would require a bureaucratic appendage at the national level larger than that needed to manage U.S. coverage.

Nor would the plan include dentistry (except as incidental to medical problems) or long-term nursing care, except for occasional high-end short stays and in hospices as is now common with Medicare. The reason for excluding dentistry, as mentioned, is that its practice is all but separate from medical care, rarely involves in-patient status, and is not a major contributor to spiraling costs. The reason for excluding long-term custodial care is almost the opposite. It is a major financial problem, but the parameters operate differently and need to be tackled from a different perspective by a different plan.

The organization at the national level would be small, and because the proposal is an outgrowth of Medicare, the staffing would likely be carved out of the present Health Services Finance Administration. However, it would be detached from the Department of Health and Human Services and set up as a quasi-independent agency analogous to the Federal Reserve Board and have its own Board of Commissioners. The vast amount of funds it would superintend, and the issues it would face continuously, would no longer warrant its being buried in a sub-cabinet level position under the thumb and whims of whoever happens to occupy the oval office.

In effect, the Board of Commissioners would oversee the operation of the second largest system in the world. Only Social Security is larger, and the overwhelming part of its operations consists of monthly checks and direct deposits to banks based on formulas prescribed by Congress, plus the keeping of Social Security records and processing of applications, again based on detailed criteria established by Congress. About the only tasks which require judgment are the adjudication of applications for disability benefits and supplementary social security payments. This explains why its administrative overhead is only one percent of its funding.

Now one of the objectives of the proposed system here is to come as close as possible to the simplicity inherent in the administration of Social Security, notwithstanding that the issues are more complex and dynamic than processing monthly checks. So to keep it simple and to endow the organization with resiliency, the idea is to vest the responsibility for shaping the resolution of those issues with the Board of Commissioners and have them negotiate directly with Congress for annual confirmation or revision of the major decisions that are legislative in nature.

Predictably, the most pressing of those issues will be: (a) the extent of coverage, (b) the scope of copayments and subsidization of the indigent, (c) sources of funding, and (d) tax or premium rates imposed on employees by way of their employers. This will require a responsive, accurate automated information system, else the proposed Board of Commissioners could do little more than make guesses. The membership of that Board would be established by Congress, but for starters the following might be considered:

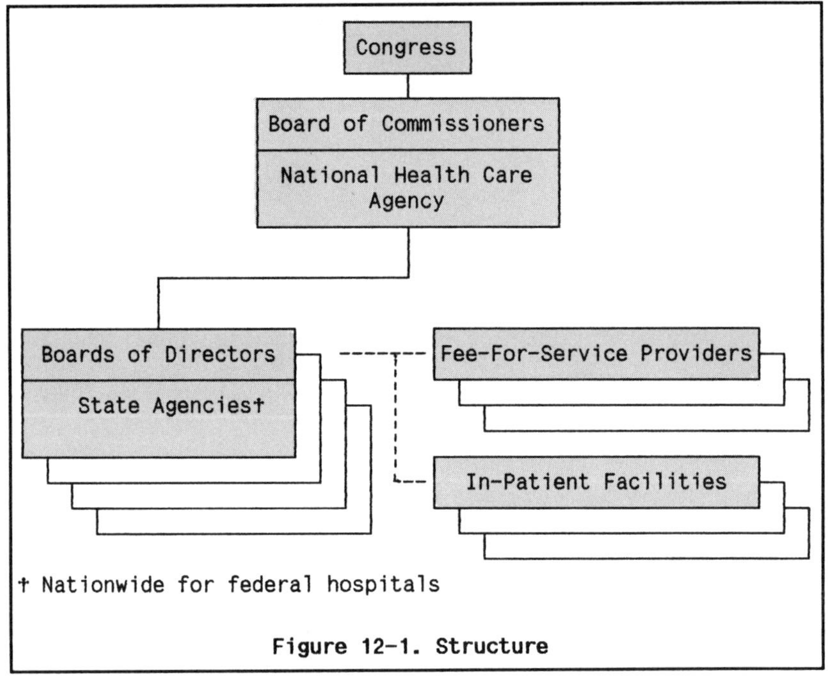

Figure 12-1. Structure

Ex Officio

- Secretary of the Department of Health & Human Services
- Executive Director of the American Medical Association
- Executive Director of the American Hospital Association
- Executive Director of the American Association of Retired Persons
- President of the American Federation of Labor-Congress of Industrial Organizations (AFL-CIO)

- Executive Director of the Consumers Union, or similar consumer group designated by Congress.
- Executive Director of the U.S. Chamber of Commerce, or similar organization designated by Congress.

Appointed

- Two individuals, one each appointed by the U.S. Senate and the U.S. House of Representative respectively (neither serving nor employed by Congress). On even-numbered years the appointee from the House would be the chairman. On odd-numbered years, the appointee of the Senate would serve in that capacity.
- Two individuals appointed by the President without the requirement for Senate confirmation.

Additionally, a jurist qualified to practice before the Supreme Court, and *perhaps* nominated by that body, should be appointed to serve as legal advisor to the Commissioners, provided said advisor had not been in active practice as advocate or jurist for at least two years preceding appointment and would not do so during tenure.

The rationale for the ex officio mix is to ensure a balanced representation of providers, payers, regulators, and spokesmen for employees and other consumers. Insurance companies are intentionally excluded as they would be competing for the business at the state level. Moreover, any individual who was or had been associated with the insurance industry at any time during the preceding three years would be ineligible for appointment and would be removed from office if such a relationship were established during tenure.

The rationale for the appointees is to ensure balanced representation from the legislative and elected executive branches of government without the squabbles that of late have evolved in various confirmation hearings. And as for the legal advisor, the intent is to ensure the presence of a jurisprudential scholar, i.e., a noted professor at a college of law. This would be important if health care is regarded as a right, however unwise that might be.

Now it is true that the ex officio members could outvote the appointees, but there are checks and balances. First, the authority to set coverage and the general index for reimbursement would remain with Congress. Second, it would take high consensus to get that mix to vote as a bloc. Third, either the total Board must seek a consensus for its annual recommendations to Congress or else leave the fate of the system to political whims. This doesn't mean Congress must buy the annual recommendations, but it does mean that if it arbitrarily or capriciously overrules them, the consumers and recipients, read voters, would perceive it instantly.

As for tenure of the appointees, a single four-year term of office, with the four appointments staggered one per year, would seem the simplest way to go about it. Turning, then, to the full-time organization at the national level, the limited responsibilities should determine its size and scope. The five major responsibilities would be:

• *Periodic Distribution of Funds.* This would be the primary function of the national-level agency and would be based on input data from the state-level agencies. In all probability, this would occur on a weekly basis and consist of adjustments to a predetermined average amount as justified by the simple but continuous reporting requirements of the state-level agencies. In return for the simplicity, however, these state agencies would be subject to detailed audit by an external agency.

• *National Practitioner Data Bank.* This function would be continued at the national level but it should be restricted to its original intent plus information on those doctors who had attempted to levy a surcharge on patients for covered services.

• *Approval of Hospital Capacity.* This is one function that could be delegated to state-level agencies but shouldn't. Those agencies are provider-oriented by design and therefore, to put the matter in diplomatic terms, might not have sufficient objectivity to fully assess the impact of increasing bed capacity. However, the state agencies would retain the authority to open standby wings (staffed as needed by the vast number of on-call (PRN) nurses) in existing hospitals to accommodate disasters and other emergencies.

• *Administrative Processing of State-Level Appeals.* Inevitably, each state agency will file numerous appeals on funding adjustments and other matters, and these must be heard under the administrative equivalent of due process. To avoid more than an occasional impasse, the lines of authority between Congress and the Board of Commissioners must be drawn carefully. The occasional unresolved issue can best be settled by a Congressional hearing, or that failing, by the courts.

• *Annual Plans and Updated Five-Year Projections.* The funding allocation for each year would have to be submitted to Congress annually, probably a half-year before the actual fiscal year begins. This would include recommendations for expanded or reduced coverage, changes to copayment schedules, the estimated cost-of-living boost to both taxes/premiums and copayments, and new sources of funding. The accompanying updated five-year projection would be intended to assess the effect of those recommendations over a longer period.

* * *

Equally important are the tasks and responsibilities to be excluded from oversight by this agency. The important ones include:

• *Investigation of Fraud or Malpractice.* Investigation of fraud should be left to the Federal Bureau of Investigation, which already has assumed a major part of that responsibility, or other federal agency that Congress may direct. As for malpractice, that should be left to the state agencies and the court systems. And as for periodic audits of the state-level agencies, this could be done by the General Accounting Office. More on this later.

• *Research.* The national-level agency would be primarily fiduciary not scholarship, hence research would be beyond its pale. The obvious exception would be on funding, coverage and copayment trade-offs, which are part and parcel of its annual recommendations to Congress.

• *Collection of Funds.* The actual collection of funds from employers and from jurisdictions and institutions in lieu of local funding of public health should remain with the Department of the Treasury and/or the Social Security Administration. The mechanisms are all in place and work well.

• *Subsidization of the Indigent.* This would be primarily a state-level function except for distribution of funds and coordinating updates to the formulas as part of he annual recommendations to Congress. The issuance of the cards should be in the state of domicile, not residence, of each individual. The one exception might be a national data bank of qualifying recipients to detect fraud and multiple applications, but this could by done by linking state databases. If a national database were established, only the Social Security number and the state and date of the current application or update need be maintained. Then each time a new application or update is filed, the individual processing it would make a quick check with the national data bank similar to the way credit card purchases are checked for canceled accounts.

STRUCTURE AT THE STATE LEVEL

The second tier is at the state level, one agency per state, plus separate agencies for administration of federal providers that may become part of the system, e.g., the VA and stateside military station hospitals. The reason for this subdivision is that it coincides with state licensing boards and court systems but makes exceptions for the federal units.

However, each state agency would require district offices for processing applications and semi-annual renewals for subsidization authorization cards. The ideal place to locate these offices would be in hospitals or clinics that bear most of this traffic and therefore would provide one-stop health care, sort of, for the indigent. However, the staff of these offices would be employees of the state agency, not the host.

Next, before delineating the specific responsibilities of these agencies, bear in mind the balancing act imposed on them. They must distribute payments to providers based on formulas and indices set nationally (adjusted for regional wage differences) while at the same time serving as an organized spokesman for providers. One way to do this would be to require each agency to have a board of seven directors, four of whom would be active providers practicing or managing health care facilities within the state.

Further, each agency would be entitled to administrative funding of a base amount plus a sliding (downward) scale percentage of its payments to providers. Within that budget, each could organize itself any way it saw fit, provided that it could meet the reporting requirements. There is no need to turn the national agency into a den mother. In more detail, the responsibilities would be:

• *Payments to Providers.* This would be on a per-diem basis to in-patient care facilities, probably twice a month adjusted for average DRG severity over the preceding six months, and straight per-service payment to other providers. The exception would be payment of salaries for employed physicians, and that should not exceed the equivalent of cumulative fees-for service. Direct payment from the national agency to hospitals is to be avoided even if it were slightly more efficient, as that would tend to undermine the authority of the state agencies.

• *Assessment of Hospital Capacity.* Requests for additional hospital capacity and perhaps major services that are not essential to all hospitals would be processed but not approved at this level. Because of the negative effect of unused capacity, and the ability of tight capacity to indirectly ration elective services, the burden of proof, so to speak, would be on the provider. The state agency would be expected to err on the side of the provider in borderline cases, but the national agency would lean the other way.

• *Subsidization of the Indigent.* As mentioned, the state agencies would administer the authorization subsystem and make payments to providers for that portion of the copayments that are subsidized. So in this one case payments to in-patient facilities would be based on the equivalent of supplementary fees cumulative for the same period as per-diem reimbursements.

GEOGRAPHICAL DISTRIBUTION

The responsibilities outlined in this chapter gloss over the problem of ensuring geographic distribution and availability of providers, which in practice refers to inner city slums and sparsely populated rural regions. That problem invites eventual intrusion on the part of the federal government trying to do good in its usual ineffective manner, so the way to approach it is with economic incentives that would encourage a better distribution but not force it. The main incentives in this regard have already been discussed at length. These include equitable per-diem reimbursement for all hospitals no matter where located, and consistent, balanced payment formulas for all covered fee-for-service practitioners. But by themselves, these provisions are insufficient to cover the waterfront.

The primary reason is that inner city slums are something of a combat zone and have the highest concentration of murders, drug pushers (and addicts), and other criminals; the least educated segment of the population and the least motivated to do anything about it; the highest concentrations of poverty and perhaps alcoholism, and in general the least favorable physical environment in which to work. For all but the most menial jobs (whose incumbents may not be in a position to go elsewhere), it takes considerable altruism to work in these areas if the same income can be made in a more pleasant suburb. Moreover, under a national plan public hospitals might close. Being strapped for cash, many cities and counties would see financial daylight by getting rid of them and substituting triage clinics and buses to transport the indigent to suburban hospitals.

Rural regions present the opposite problem. Many offer a pristine beauty, but the population of the seventeen least populous states is about equal to the Los Angeles metropolitan area (16 million). When the larger cities in those states are factored out of the equation, the number of states increases to 30 states.[1] Another statistic is that the least populated geographical half of the United States claims less than two percent of its population. Building comprehensive hospitals and locating medical specialists within a short driving distance for each resident in these areas is clearly impractical. The best that can be done is to encourage more family practitioners to work there, and even at that, some would have to ride circuit continuously.

A few rural communities subsidize the medical education of a doctor in return for his or her practicing in that area for a stipulated number of years. A variation of this is used by the government with some medical education loans. The recipient is obliged to serve in a designated specialty or area for a specified number of years in return for cancelling the loan, with the face value of the loan tripling for noncompliance. Unfortunately, these measures have not yielded the providers necessary and the latter is poorly enforced.

It's an intricate problem, but two simple measures could make a real dent in it. First, both urban slum and rural regions could be zoned into three categories: A = severe need, and B = moderate need, and C = borderline. Fees and salaries (computed as a percent of the per-diem reimbursement for hospitals) could be increased 15 percent for the A zone, 10 percent for B, and 5 percent for C, for services physically provided in those zones. If each zone had 5 percent of the population, that would mean a 1.5 percent increase overall (15% * 5/100 + 10% * 5/100 + 5% *5/100 = 1.5%). To pay for this, reimbursements elsewhere would be reduced by 1.5 percent.

The second measure would be to tax all political subdivisions for a fair share of health care costs equal on average to that which they now provide. The revenue would be added to the general fund and redistributed in the form of per-diem payments to public hospitals the same as private ones. That is, having paid for them in part, and being guaranteed higher-than-normal reimbursement, these jurisdictions would have a major incentive to keep them open.

The last point to discuss here is copayment. The electorate would not be thrilled if the poor were granted excessive subsidization while they, especially the lower income consumer units, had to bear the copayments in full. On many occasions, this would result in lower net income than the poor received without working for it. So the criteria for subsidization should be tight not loose, and perhaps subdivided into four categories: 25 percent subsidization, 50 percent, 75 percent, and full, renewed every 6 months.

FRAUD AND MALPRACTICE

Notwithstanding some fine legal arguments that can be marshaled to the contrary, fraud is a felony with well-defined criteria that should be prosecuted in the criminal court system. By contrast, malpractice, except in cases of wanton negligence, is largely a civil matter. Moreover, malpractice (in the legal sense) ranges from might be called the learning curve experienced by dedicated residents to stuporous incompetence or worse.

True, the definitions of fraud vary, but most of those variations revolve around "an intentional perversion of truth for the purpose of inducing another in reliance upon it to part with some valuable thing belonging to him or to surrender a legal right."[2] In terms of health care, this includes every instance of a fee-for-service provider filing a claim for a service that he or she did not provide, or alternatively filing a claim for a more expensive service than the one actually provided. In terms of hospital claims, at least under the system proposed in this book, fraud would consist of intentionally falsifying DRG data in order to obtain a higher per-diem reimbursement than earned or a failure to deduct patient days for non-covered services.

Fraud does not include claims for services rendered beyond the needs of the patient, even when the practice is obviously based on greed. As mentioned, doctors who own or control certain laboratories have been found to order tests four times more frequently than those who don't.[3] That is a serious problem and the cost of it may even exceed outright fraud, but it cannot be dealt with in the same way. It is not a crime, per se. Accordingly, this proposal advocates draconian measures to reduce and punish fraudulent claims and then takes a different tack with respect to malpractice and what some analysts erroneously call "soft fraud." And keep in mind that there is a relationship between some excess services and malpractice. Many doctors order additional tests as a defense against possible suits.

The one common element to these two approaches would be the fee-for-service claims form. It would consist of a single page printed on one side only, which could be submitted electronically. For most services, only the top half would be filled in. The bottom half would be for reporting unusual conditions. But copies of these claims would be maintained in an image processing system at state-level agencies and reviewed periodically for patterns of fraud and wantonly excessive services with respect to needs. As mentioned in chapter 8, this technique is used with increasing frequency and success, especially by insurance companies, to detect statistical aberrations insofar as they correlate with wrongdoing. The measures to be taken against fraud, then, would be:

• *Investigation and Prosecution by a Federal Agency.* A fee-for-service provider that was suspected of fraudulent claims or even attempting to file them would be investigated by the FBI, provided the case against the individual, partnership, or corporation was substantial. This is not a witch hunt.

• *Suspension of Reimbursement for Fee-for-Service Providers.* Any provider convicted of fraud would have all reimbursement suspended for one-year for the first offense, three years for the second, and for life after the third. It is tempting to substitute suspension of their licenses to practice but this would be undue interference in the prerogatives of other agencies, and it would be moot anyway. Without reimbursement, the license to practice, except perhaps for vanity-market plastic surgeons and those few physicians who have indentured themselves to the wealthy, would be meaningless.

• *Involvement by Clerical Personnel.* Any clerk or other employee of a fee-for-service provider who knowingly participated in the submission of a fraudulent claim would also be tried and if found guilty fined a minimum of $10,000 per offense. However, any such employee who was ordered to do this, but refused to do so, and reported the attempt to federal authorities would be paid $100,000 tax free upon conviction of the perpetrator. This may sound excessive but in practice many crimes are prosecuted as a result of paid informants, and in this case the idea is not to pay informants but to make fraudulent claims so risky that few if any providers would make the attempt. Moreover, this reporting option would be limited to outright fraud, not billing for questionable or excess services actually rendered or provided, and the employee would have had to have been ordered knowingly to participate in the felony.

• *Hospital Administrators.* When a hospital administrator intentional falsifies DRG or other data in order to increase the hospital's per-diem reimbursement, then upon conviction in federal court, he or she would be fined a minimum of $50,000 and the hospital another $100,000 for the first offense and $250,000 for the second offense, regardless if it was committed by the same or a different administrator. In addition, the per-diem reimbursement to any hospital would cease in totality for that period of time it employed in any capacity an administrator convicted twice for fraud.

So much for crime. As mentioned, malpractice and questionable or excess services are another matter. It has been said that every doctor in training kills a few patients before he earns his spurs. By this is meant that in critical cases, he or she may err slightly on the side of too much intervention and thus cause the patient to expire sooner than would have occurred in the natural course of events.

And there are even more cases where a timely accurate diagnosis is impractical and therefore the treatment rendered may later prove damaging if not fatal.

Further, the practice of basing the judgment on "what a reasonably competent physician would have done in a similar case" is also flawed because perfectly competent doctors will not always do the same thing in the same circumstances. If they did, the practice of medicine could be reduced to computer software and computer-guided laser surgery, so the measures to be taken or not taken against malpractice would be:

• *No Damage Limitations.* The idea of limiting damages is interesting, but in point of fact most of the high awards arise from flagrant malpractice and they do serve as a warning to others. Moreover, the majority of Congressmen are lawyers. They would not warm to such a measure.

• *Published Criteria.* The idea of specifying procedures and tests essential to prove a lack of malpractice may be a better idea. This is akin to prescribed protocols and DRGs, but the emphasis would be reducing unnecessary services, not controlling the length of inpatient stays.

• *Prohibited Ownership of Unnecessary Ancillaries.* No fee-for-service provider should be permitted to have any financial interest or effective control in any ancillary that wasn't essential for his or her trade. With few exceptions, there is little justification for a practicing physician to own or control laboratories. If he does, then he should concentrate on running the lab and stay out of patient practice per se. This would also extend to ownership of long-term nursing care facilities unless the practice was limited to its patients. But it would not extend to non-controlling shares on the stock market and certainly not to mutual funds.

• *Published Information.* Every hospital that had one or more physicians or other practitioners on its staff who, exclusive of cases incurred while a resident, had been found guilty of malpractice in a civil proceeding, or who otherwise settled out of court in an amount exceeding $2,000, three or more times in the preceding five years would be required to publish a monthly updated list of such doctors with summary information on each case, and provide a copy of the current list to every patient admitted. The temptation would be to reduce the number to two cases in a three rather than a five year period, but the chance of making two honest mistakes is still significant. Three cases would remove the doubt.

13

DEVELOPMENT

*Which of you, intending to build a tower, sitteth not down first
and counteth the cost, whether he hath sufficient to finish it.*
                                                        - Luke 14:28

The usual route for reform in the United States is to impose a grand solution
by fiat and then hope it works out. Accordingly, many fail and many others fall
short of expectations. This is because the solution often ignores facts, data and
the dynamics imposed by those realities. On the other hand, experimenting with
$750 billion worth of services for a few years is impractical. So the only possible
solution is to build a model and work with that. To the extent it accurately mimics
what it purports to model is the extent to which it can prove useful.

True, there are caveats when it comes to health care models. First, the
providers themselves must take an interest and participate in the development
and operation. Second it must be resilient enough to capture the main operating
factors in all of their potential combinations. Third, the model itself should have
the capability of evolving into the prototype financial management tool for the
intended system. That's a tall order, yet seven years ago the Director for the
Office of Management and Budget in the office of the President maintained the
entire national budget on a small laptop computer with only enough memory to
hold the equivalent of 24 pages of text.[1] Today's automation technology has
advanced a hundred-fold beyond that relic and offers the opportunity to model
just about any system at bargain basement prices.

ECONOMIC PARAMETERS

Roughly speaking, the term parameter means a factor, the value of which
determines the limits of a system. The term was coined in mathematics and the
system it referred to was a system or set of equations. Yet because anything
dynamic can be described with equations, the term osmosed its way into many
practical applications, especially economics. Moreover, as in mathematics, any
system can have more than one parameter. Another way of thinking about

parameters is in terms of leverage, or how pressure at a few critical points can exert exceptional influence on a system. In this sense, the concept coincides with terms adopted earlier in this book, namely centers of gravity and interior lines. It is time, then, to review the dynamics of these parameters.

To start, the governing parameters are: (a) the main source of funding, which would be a tax or premium imposed on employers in proportion to employees and wages plus, as at present, premiums charged against Social Security benefits for retirees, (b) additional sources of funding, to include shifting of funding for agencies that would no longer be needed and by way of disincentive taxes on unhealthy substances, (c) the costs and billings of providers, which depend on the scope of coverage in the system, and (d) copayment on the part of recipients, which to some extent must be subsidized for the indigent or what is the same, paying providers directly for all or part for some copayments. To these, the model should have built-in incentives to encourage a better geographical distribution of providers in inner cities and rural regions.

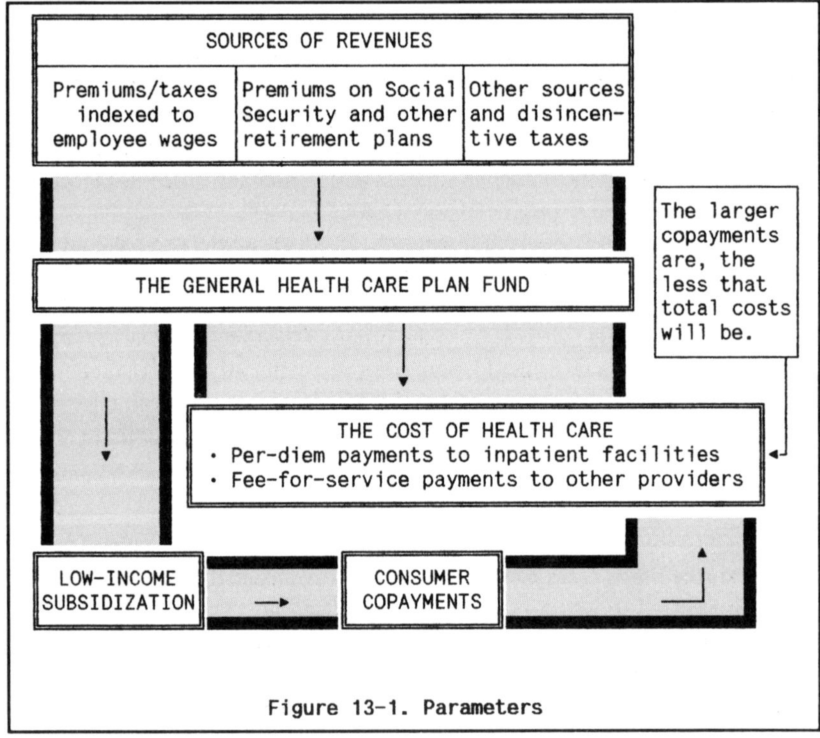

Figure 13-1. Parameters

Figure 13-1 illustrates the relationships among these parameters. If the funding is increased, either more services can be provided or the providers can be paid more for the same services or a mixture of both. The same is true if copayments are increased, not only in absolute dollars but because that would serve as a disincentive to use available services for minor ailments and the incessant begging for tranquilizer prescriptions to escape life's problems.

It should also be noted that costs per hospital day would drop significantly on a *one-time basis* if excess hospital capacity were shut down and the high costs of claims processing virtually eliminated. Just how much would take some analysis, but the median could easily be factored into the model. Similarly, the capping of fee-for-service charges would also lower the total bill.

So much for the internal dynamics. This being a democracy, the system would experience continuous pressure to expand coverage, reduce payments to providers, reduce copayments, and/or increase subsidization of low-income consumers once in operation. But if the system is set up on a self-pay basis—admittedly rare in government today—then every attempt to do so could be countered immediately (in hours) with the consequences in financial terms.

However, one point needs emphasis. Projections of future costs are always based on probability. Probabilities vary. If someone falls from an aircraft in flight without a parachute, there's a 99.9999 percent chance he won't survive. (A rare few have lived to tell about it, one by landing on a steep snow field.) By contrast, the outcome of a twenty-foot fall is much less certain. Thus any projection of future net costs must be considered to be a median value. To the extent it is more uncertain, that value must be hedged with plus-or-minus data.

PHASING

Not surprisingly, the development of models often fall prey to the same mistakes made when an attempt is made to impose reform without thinking through the consequences. Accordingly, many systems developers recognize that two or three models in succession may be necessary. The first edition almost always fails. There are too many details and relationships that cannot be foreseen, but the experience gained with that first edition can lead to a more workable second edition.

That too will probably fall short of the mark, yet it will usually work well enough to more fully experiment with the intended objectives. Finally, with those lessons learned and if carefully built, the third edition has a good chance of succeeding. Figure 13-2 illustrates this phasing, although it does not graphically relate the amount of time spent on each phase nor the scope of detail to be tested.

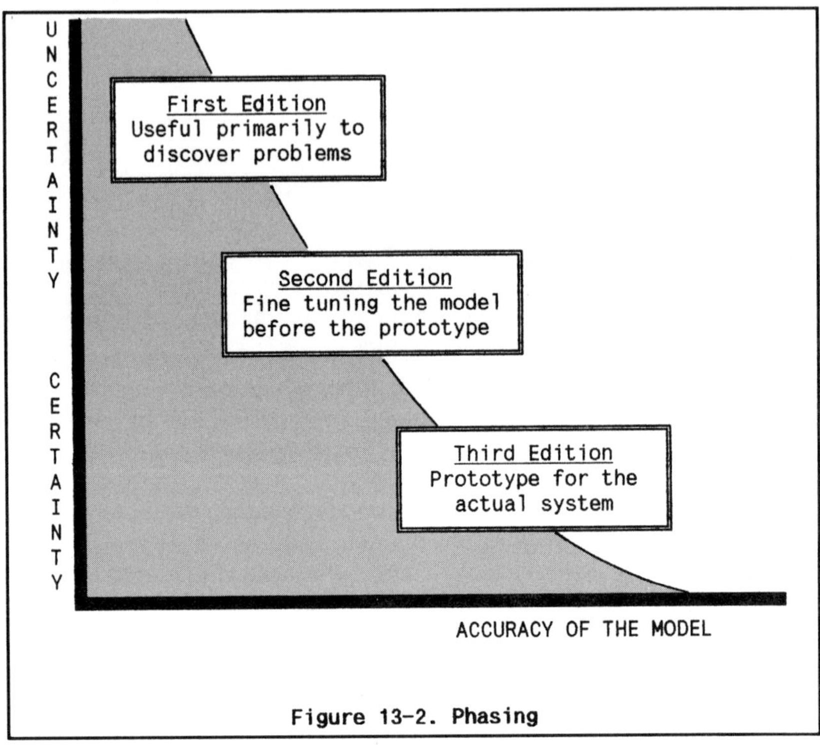

Figure 13-2. Phasing

Now building a model can be time consuming and building three of them would be a major undertaking. On the other hand, the idea is to explore relationships and identify major gaps, so the first one should be built on the run, so to speak, making maximum use of what is called productivity software, in this case a spreadsheet. Productivity software lets the user concentrate on what needs to be analyzed or done while automating the tedious work common to programming a requirement from scratch. Pushed to the limit, models developed with this kind of software can be finished in a week or less, sometimes in a matter of hours. So before going into the scope for each phase it would be well to review the bidding on spreadsheets.

Spreadsheets are automated ledgers. The popularity of these automated ledgers in the business world is confirmed by the more than twenty million licensed copies in use. At least five popular versions from different software publishers are available, of which the one offered by the Lotus Development Corporation has the lion's share of the market. But how can a ledger operate as a decision support system? Because, in this case, the decisions that need to be supported all have a financial bottom line to assess, and automated ledgers can be used to generate and analyze thousands of different combinations. Moreover, they can be networked, nationwide if necessary, to simulate a far flung organization, and combined with interactive processing. The latter, in part, means that whenever factors or parameters are changed in one part of a model, all other parts of the model dependent on that change are instantly updated.

Of special interest are three additional features available on many versions of the software. The first is called a *three-dimensional spreadsheet*. This means that several hundred spreadsheets can be integrated into one file. Moreover, any one of those spreadsheets can automatically draw data from other files including updates to that source data. In practical terms, then, if one spreadsheet is used to represent each state-level agency (or equivalent) then the first spreadsheet in the set would represent the total. Every change to any element in any state would instantly be reflected in both the ledger for that state and in the national-level ledger. Vice-versa, if there were any change to funding levels, the effect on each state would display instantly on that state's ledger.[2] Figure 13-3 depicts how this can be done.

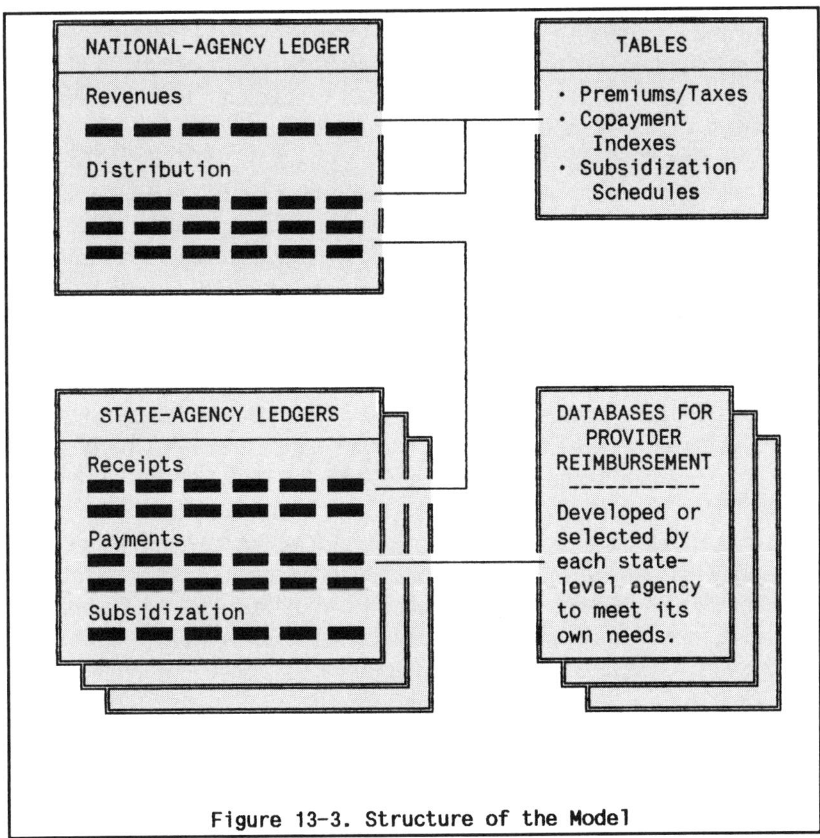

Figure 13-3. Structure of the Model

This does introduce the problem of keeping track of the effect from all of these changes. Not to worry. The second feature solves the problem. Every step of the analysis can be saved to a different file without affecting the original, a technique which is sometimes called *templating*. Moreover, yet another spreadsheet can be used to compare the results of these specific analyses, all by automatic file linking.

The third feature is the ability to write miniature programs (called *macros*) into a spreadsheet which can then further automate the experimental variation of different factors and then instantly display before-and-after graphs of the results. Too good to be true? Not really. The technique is so pervasive in business that its practitioners have earned the sobriquet "spreadsheet jockeys."

To continue, then, the first edition of this application would experiment with the computer model for a month or so in a single location using a local area network and several computers. This would permit simultaneous access by multiple users. The objectives would be: (a) to gain a better understanding of the dynamics among the main parameters, (b) to develop rough estimates of the total costs that the national agency would have to fund, and (c) to identify the main sticking points between the national agency and the state-level agencies, at least in terms of data exchange. At the state-level simulation, input data would be estimated "manually" and entered directly on its spreadsheet.

The second edition would be more complex and use files or subordinate spreadsheets to represent providers. These provider files would harness the capability of the software to work as if it were a database. The numerical totals on them would then be automatically linked to the state roll-up spreadsheet. As a matter of practical concern, the operation of this model should still be limited to one physical location, but it can be dispersed into several rooms and manned by provider representatives. Further, the development of this second edition should be done by an independent group of technicians who observe but do not actively participate in the first. The reasons are: (a) it overlaps the time required for both editions, and (b) it would lower the temptation to simply modify the first edition instead building a better one from scratch.

After six months or so of experimentation with the second edition, work can start on the third. This time, however, the model would be operated on a wide area network with stations in at least five to seven states and the balance simulated at the central location. The spreadsheet software would still work for the exchange of data between the nation and state agencies, but the mass of data required at the state levels would require a separate database application.

Moreover, only the exchange of information between the national agency and the state agencies is to be standardized. How each of the latter build and run their system beyond that is their business, provided the data can be audited by an independent agency. So the third edition should employ a variety of state-level systems. Then when and if implemented, each state could: (a) choose one of them, (b) select but modify one, or (c) build one from scratch.

Two final caveats. First, when it comes to computer systems, the normal tendency of the government is to avoid prototypes and instead go directly to detailed specifications and planning.[3] When exceptions are made for very large systems that have many unknowns, then even the prototype is subjected to massive bureaucratic administration that can consume years. And because overcoming or bypassing that obstacle would be nearly impossible, the alternative is for some non-government agency to take the initiative and just do it. The cost, at least for the first edition, would be negligible.

Second, if the providers take the initiative for the planning and development, their interests will be more firmly anchored in the final product. Else the experience of increasing federal intrusion into professional prerogatives over the last ten years should leave no doubt that the tourniquet will be tightened further as the costs continue to outdistance the available revenues. Enough said.

14

PERSPECTIVE

The human struggle for a way to live without work will
finally test the strength of our institutions.

         - Abraham Lincoln

The proposal outlined in this book aims at providing adequate health care services for every person within the country and controlling the expense of those services, at least sufficiently to cover the cost of the additional coverage. It would do this by eliminating excess hospital capacity plus the high cost of insurance overhead and the bulk of claims processing administration. It would also cap reimbursements for all fee-for-service bills and effectively prohibit excess charges, at least for covered services. However, those covered services would not include dentistry or long-term nursing home care. The latter is an especially troubling problem, but it is a different beast and must be approached in a different way.

The mechanics are a streamlined version of the present Medicare system. The key is a general fund that would draw revenue from a number of sources but primarily a tax or premium on every employee plus a premium levied against Social Security payments. That fund would then be distributed to state-level agencies that would reimburse fee-for-service providers directly and hospitals on a much simplified per-diem rather than a per case basis. Services of every kind would require immediate copayment on the part of individuals receiving them, but the indigent and the poor would be subsidized to the extent of their bona fide poverty. The plan would also call for certain economic incentives to encourage providers to practice in inner city slums and sparse rural regions.

The key word there is "encourage," because while this plan emphasizes economic incentives to achieve its purposes, the undertow is that of restoring a sense of professionalism to the practice of medicine, a sense that is being eroded by the increasing intrusion of federal auditors and other authorities into the prerogatives of doctors, hospitals, and other providers. That is, while the proposal tackles cost and distribution problems head-on, it would also put more distance between Washington and the operating room.

This would be accomplished by reliance on "the law of averages" to control costs, primarily by way of closing down excess hospital capacity, perhaps even more than that in order to indirectly ration some elective procedures. Then it would finance hospitals on a average-cost-per-day basis, adjusted for regional wage differentials and for average patient load severity. There would no longer be any insurance claims for hospitalization, except when filing for subsidized copayments for the poor and the indigent.

Similarly, physicians would be reimbursed for claims without question initially, but the claim would be limited to a national schedule adjusted for regional differentials, and no surcharges would be permitted. However, the pattern of claims for each provider would be audited by automated decision support systems to detect patterns of fraud and excessive-care claims relative to the nature of the dysfunctions treated.

The proposal also emphasizes resiliency. Its internal administrative lines are about the simplest that can be devised and still accommodate the vast range of practitioners in the country. The national-level agency could be operated with only a few hundred staff, and the state-level agencies would be much smaller than, say, an existing Blue Cross-Blue Shield agency in a large metropolitan city. Moreover, the plan would have the ability to instantly project the costs of adding additional services or reducing copayments, or, alternatively, to project the savings from curtailing coverage or increasing copayment.

In short, the proposal attempts to give first priority to the ethical centers of gravity for health care, namely to make it available, physically and financially, to all who need it, but at the same time paying careful attention to economic realities. Those realities translate to a conservative menu of coverage and significant copayments. Even when the poor are subsidized, it still means a reasonable sharing of costs and a continuous review of eligibility.

This is not to say that the proposal is without its shortcomings. Far from it, and it doesn't have a ghost of chance of being adopted in the immediate future. The reason is that for the moment at least, the supposed crisis in health care is more political hype than reality for the majority of voters. Eventually, the accelerating costs will infect that majority but not this year, or next year, or perhaps the year after that. As such, the providers, especially insurance companies and not a few physicians, will do whatever is necessary to keep milking the existing system legally for as long as possible.

Even if the crisis stage had been reached, any proposal must contend with the inertia of all infrastructure toward change. Harvey's discovery of circulation of the blood was ignored for 30 years, and the finding by Oliver Wendell Holmes Sr., MD, (father of the famed Supreme Court Justice) that unsanitary conditions in hospitals infected patients more than the services help cure them went unheeded for 15 or 20 years. Or a proposal might suffer the fate of the Gregorian calendar. The need to correct the deficiency in the Julian calendar was recognized by the Council of Nicea in A.D. 730. After 742 years of review, the Vatican agreed. The details were worked out for another 140 years, and a subsequent pontiff, Pope Gregory, promulgated the new calendar in the year 1582. It was accepted immediately by the Papal States, but the rest of the world took its time. Russia was the last major country to go along, coinciding with the Bolshevik Revolution in 1917. Total elapsed time: 1,187 years.

It would be nice if that were the only obstacle, but any reform of health care must also face up to a more insidious problem, and that is the condition and mindset into which the country has sunk. This degradation has evolved slowly since the close of World War II and is now so ingrained that nothing sort of an extreme crisis could reverse it. The litany has been cited by numerous writers, from scholars to Lee Iacocca.1 And, of course, it has been ignored. It's not so much a matter of "crying from the wilderness" as recalling Plato's description of the men chained up in the den and suddenly seeing their own shadows by way of a light behind them.2 They didn't take kindly to the disturbance, and ever since disturbers of this genre have earned an unprintable nickname.

And what is this litany? In a pessimistic moment one might conclude that the elected administrations over the past 20 years have simply grown irrelevant, at least when it comes to domestic affairs; that Congress has become encrusted with itself and bent on reelection primarily by way by doling out more and bigger handouts, notwithstanding the astronomical national debt; that the Supreme Court has become something of jurisprudential yo-yo, what with decisions on critical issues alternating between 5-4 votes then 4-5 votes (and not a trace of the likes of a Holmes, a Brandeis. or a Frankfurtur seen in years); and of journalism that seems willing to sell the soul of its irreplaceable role in a democracy in return for a few tidbits dropped by elected officials.

Then, too, there is the matter of the easily documented decline of morals and ethics in every sector of public and private life, coupled with an increasing willingness to tolerate it. Every year, between $100 and $120 billion in income tax liability goes unpaid. Twenty billion of that alone is an attempt to conceal wages reported on W-2 forms. Worse, 23 percent of the population feels it is perfectly all right to defraud automobile insurance companies with false claims to compensate for premiums paid in past years or to cover the deductible. To this must be added the accelerating crime and drug addict rates and perhaps another dozen sources of dry rot that permeate every joist of the civil infrastructure. In all fairness to critics, however, it must be stated that in some quarters the foregoing perspective would be considered optimistic.

What is important? It isn't education. Probably less than half the country can read and understand anything but the simplest piece of serious writing, and 20 percent seem to have trouble reading a stop sign. No, the important things, as measured in time and dollars invested, are sports, soap operas and television in general, lotteries, and accumulating as much personal debt as possible. One longs for the day when television was merely a vast wasteland. Then there is the emphasis on highly emotionally charged issues such as capital punishment, vivisection, and the various conspiracy theories on who killed John F. Kennedy.

It is also a matter of pumping governments at all levels for as many free and subsidized services as can be had. This trend has progressed to the point where the country has become addicted to welfare in all of its many forms and which increasingly regards personal responsibility as an interesting but archaic theory. Dictators drive their countries to destruction; free-wheeling democracies vote for it.

And so to this paradigm, some form of subsidization of health insurance will be added within the next few years. This can only serve to increase the national debt beyond the point of manageable return and perhaps set the stage for a variation on socialism where the government begins to guarantee every human need as a right. Strangely, that may bring about the country's renaissance. Not socialism, but the depression any further welfare will likely trigger. Addicts tend to come to their senses, if they come at all, only after they hit absolute rock bottom, when it dawns on them that the choice is to change or to accept death, spiritual or physical. Hence, a depression might bring about the recognition that the ability of the federal government to solve domestic problems is limited. It can mandate certain reforms at a macro level, but it cannot manage, much less change human nature.

Interestingly and second only to scripture, a recent survey determined that the book most often cited as an influence on reader's lives was Ayn Rand's *Atlas Shrugged*. In that book, the country tailspins into a depression and of necessity the power brokers draft the best of the Detroit industrialists to serve as benevolent dictator until the crisis abates. But if that turns out to be an accurate prophecy, it won't usher in the millennium. There are even more massive problems in the wings. Among them are the challenges of feeding the exploding world population on a planet that simply doesn't have the ability to do so beyond a certain point, especially with waste products causing a global warming trend and destroying the ozone layer at the same time.

Then there is the matter of thermonuclear technology as it spreads and eventually becomes the weapon of choice for terrorism. One must recognize that terrorists, especially those emanating from the Middle East, are fanatics and some of them would have no compunctions about using these weapons to further political causes no matter what the consequences are for themselves.

Another interesting scenario pits a rejuvenated Russia, an economically unified Western Europe, the Japanese-controlled Pacific basin, and a resurgent China in a long-term economic war with the United States, especially while the latter clings to her quaint notions on free trade. If you think not, then perhaps you should visit Hawaii and observe how Japan has taken effective control of that state. Then visit Perth, Australia, where the same process is just getting under way. Japan has much too small of a land mass to sustain her 124 million population, and Australia looks inviting indeed. They are working hard to develop cheap solar powered ocean water desalinization plants with which to turn vast deserts into farm land, and for which Australia is the obvious candidate for implementation. That country is nearly as large as the U.S. but its population is only a thirteenth of Japan's and its economic clout a mere tenth.

The point to this diatribe is that the United States, notwithstanding the recent decline and fall of the Soviet Union, will soon enough be confronted with a full slate of awesome issues. Dealing successfully with these issues depends on economic strength. That strength is not to be gained by begging for a depression. And so perhaps the recognition of the pending melee might lend sobriety to the decision making on national health care. The latter perforce is an economic watershed in a worldwide flood plain. Stay tuned.

APPENDICES

Appendix A.

APPENDIX A. NATIONAL DEBT PROJECTIONS

*Any government, like any family, can for a time, spend
more than it earns. But you and I know that a continuance of
that habit means the poor house.*

        - Franklin D. Roosevelt

The national debt is edging towards four trillion dollars, and the annual deficits are running at 300 billion dollars or more per year. Hence it is just a matter of time before the cumulative deficits increase that debt to the point where the interest on it alone will consume the annual budget. For two other reasons, that moment will come sooner than later. First, the current recession seems to have staying power and the government's reaction to it is to pour even more money into the economy, money that can be obtained only by increasing the debt. Second, a good part of the deficits are being funded with the temporary surplus in the Social Security trust fund.

This surplus results from the FICA tax being much higher than needed for immediate benefits. However, the aging population means that the annual cost of those benefits will continue to rise steeply over the next thirty to forty years, with fewer and fewer workers, proportionally speaking, to fund them. That surplus, if wisely invested, would cushion that long-term deficit, at least for the next several generations. But the investment of choice, in this case, has been the Treasury Department. Every dollar collected above benefits paid is invested in the federal government itself. In theory, there is no greater security. When the Treasury can no longer pay its debts, the security of any other investment would be moot.

In colloquial terms, Uncle Sam has deep pockets. Unfortunately, those deep pockets are empty. When the cost of the annual benefits rises to the point where it equals the annual FICA tax, the money lent to the Treasury must be repaid. But there would be no money on hand to pay it back. So it would have to borrow money from new sources in order to pay that debt plus borrow enough additional funds to cover the amount it presently "borrows" from the Social Security trust fund every year.

That's simple enough in theory, but there isn't enough money floating around to do it. Therefore the government would have to raise taxes by a large percentage or cut benefits by an equally large amount. That would depress the economy further and hence reduce revenues. In turn, that would exacerbate the pressing need to borrow more money, and so forth and so on in a vicious cycle.

To be sure, a near-miracle might occur. The country may suddenly reverse its fortunes and initiate a spectacular rate of growth for the gross domestic product. That in turn would vastly increase revenues enough to wipe out the annual deficits plus accumulate enough of a surplus to pay off the debt. Alternatively, Japanese investors could trade up from their golf course at Pebble Beach on the Monterey peninsula and buy the Brooklyn Bridge for 4 trillion dollars. The odds of either happening are about the same.

In a word, the national economy is running on fumes, and the impact of this mounting debt on health care should be obvious. If the economy is headed for a major depression, how can it possibly afford a national system, especially one that fails to control costs. Even if a plan were adopted that all but eliminated insurance overhead costs and excess hospital capacity, and capped all bona fide reimbursements, the subsidization of health care for the poor and the indigent would eat up most of those savings. Then when the pressure comes to include more services, especially long-term care, and to reduce copayments and bail out the indigent even further, the debt would soar past its present stratospheric height. Let us, then, review the bidding on basic economics.

Economics 101 teaches that when an individual or business accumulates more debt than they can pay back, they will go bankrupt unless someone else buys them out. In effect, that also applies to countries, witness the absorption of East Germany by West Germany. Most observers labeled this as a political reunification, but in economic terms it was a buy-out. West Germany got the land and its people in return for bailing them out of their de facto bankruptcy. Since the United States doesn't have any buyers in the wing, this leaves only bankruptcy if the debt cannot be paid off.

Many economists, especially those under the employ or thumb of the administration, regard that "if" as theoretical. They reason that $3.6 trillion divided among the country's 260 million people comes to roughly $13,850 apiece, much less than the average annual wage. Thus, so goes the theory, the country has mortgaged the future only in terms of months, not generations. That would be a comforting thought except for the fact it is riddled with error.

First, only about a third of the population works on a full-time equivalent basis. The rest are children growing up, retirees, and adult dependents outside the workforce. Second, debt can be repaid only from surplus, not from funds essential to keep an individual, a family, or a business going. Third, only a minority of wage earners have any significant surplus. And, fourth, the debt keeps growing at pace three to four times faster than the economy.

In practical terms, then, only the upper 30 percent or so of the population is in any position to repay the debt, and that percentage must be subdivided into tax-paying units of roughly three members per consumer unit. A consumer unit includes singles, unmarried individuals with dependents, and families. The 30 percent mark itself is based on the fact that the lower half of consumer units have no surplus income, and for the next 20 percent, the surplus is negligible.[1] In practical terms, then, when the national debt is parceled out to the upper 30 percent of the consumer units, each share comes to $138,461, and that can be repaid only from surplus, read higher taxes. Table A-1 and the accompanying graph projects the increase in that share over the next ten years, assuming a continued annual deficit of $300 billion.

The formula adds the annual deficit (increased by a factor of five percent to cover "inflation" in government) to the current debt, adding six percent interest on the amount of that debt that exceeds $3.6 trillion. That amount is divided by one-third of 30 percent of the population (which is increased by a growth rate of three percent). It does not include funding for additional health care benefits (although that is indicated on figure A-1). Also, this projection assumes that the IOU to the Social Security trust fund will not fall due within the next ten years.

Now it should be obvious that before the astronomical figures for 2002 are reached, the economy will collapse. "Not really," argue the government economists, "laws and procedures have been enacted to prevent the stock market from collapsing as it did in 1929, which have been strengthened as a result of the mini-crash that occurred in October 1987." Perhaps so, but the stock market has very little to do with it, and times have changed radically since 1929.

At the time, the economy of the country was based primarily on manufacturing and farming, the national debt was insignificant, and the trade balance, what little there was of it, was positive. The collapse of the stock market—the consequence of perceived inflated stock prices—reduced the availability of investment capital to a trickle. Banks, which held much of the stock, no longer had the assets to lend. Thus, in a chain reaction, companies went out of business or at least pared down, and that threw millions of employees out of work and reduced wages for the vast majority of the balance. Farming (and ranching) continued, but the economy could no longer pay current prices so it too suffered. The federal programs initiated by the Roosevelt administration starting in 1933 succeeded in overcoming the worst aspects of that period, but many if not most historians argue that the depression lingered until the country's participation in World War II turned the tide for good.

Now defense analysts have a saying that military planners concentrate on winning the last war. This means they ignore changes and differences in factors, hence when the next war comes, the plans stumble and sometimes fail outright. Perhaps the same is true for economic planners. For starters, even if the government were to freeze stock market prices, the public perception of the value of stock would still collapse and few would buy stock at prices that were

Table A-1. Projected Deficits

Year	Annual Deficit	Excess Interest	Cumulative Debt Total	Per Unit
1992	————————	————————	$3,600,000,000,000	$138,416
1993	$315,000,000,000	$18,900,000,000	3,933,900,000,000	146,897
1994	330,750,000,000	39,879,000,000	4,304,529,000,000	156,055
1995	347,288,000,000	63,109,000,000	4,714,925,000,000	165,955
1996	364,652,000,000	88,775,000,000	5,168,352.000,000	176,616
1997	382,884,000,000	117,074,000,000	5,668,311,000,000	188,059
1998	402,029,000,000	148,220,000,000	6,218,560,000,000	200,306
1999	422,130,000,000	182,441,000,000	6,823,131,000,000	213,378
2000	443,237,000,000	219,982,000,000	7,486,350,000,000	227,300
2001	465,398,000,000	261,105,000,000	8,212,853,000,000	242,095
2002	488,668,000,000	306,091,000,000	9,007,613,000,000	257,789

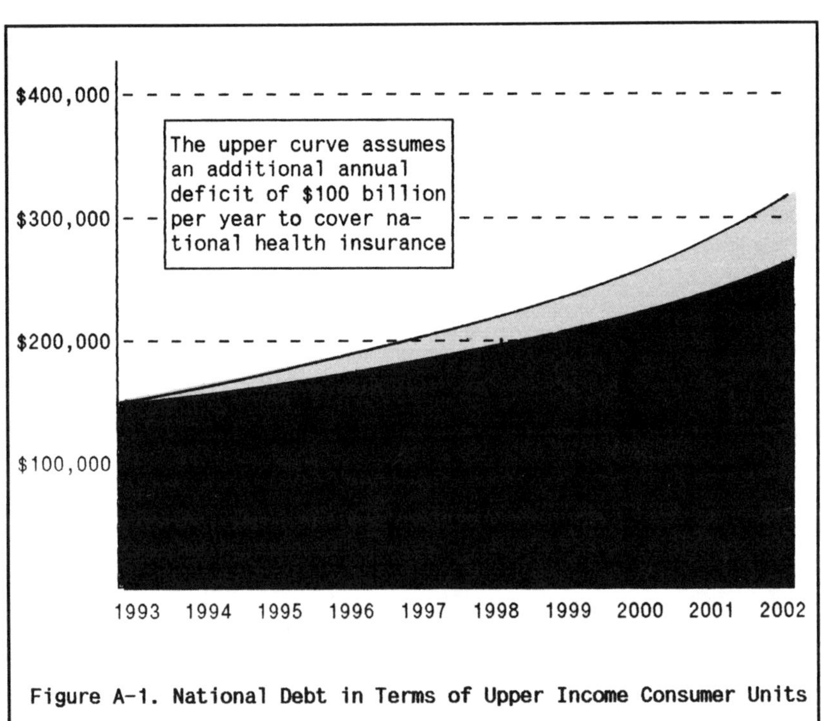

Figure A-1. National Debt in Terms of Upper Income Consumer Units

considered to be inflated. More importantly, if the companies involved—the majority of which are concentrated in the service sector not manufacturing—lose business, the dividends would fall if not evaporate. That means banks, pension funds, insurance companies, and other holders would no longer receive the income they planned on. It doesn't take wizardry to project the consequences.

But let us view the situation in more down-to-earth terms. As mentioned, the economy is service not manufacturing based. The significance is that while it is impractical for an individual to make a car for himself, he can learn to repair one and keep it longer. He can also paint his house and take care of his own children instead of sending them to a daycare center, especially when one spouse within a marriage loses his or her job.

Thus as a recession metastasizes into a depression, people out of work can no longer afford the services offered by the service sector or worse (in terms of the national economy) they no longer need them. So as the demand for these services drops, the suppliers will go out of business or at least curtail it. That means lower profits, which in turn mean lower taxes paid into the federal treasury. As taxes shrink, so too do government services, just when demand for them on the part of the newly unemployed increases. Also, the government itself will be forced to lay off employees, and that in turn would add to the demands and further reduce the tax take.

The alternative is to reduce benefits, including social security, military and civil service retirement, Medicare, unemployment compensation, and welfare programs. Fine. Most of that is taxable, or at least taxable in part, so revenues would be reduced just the same. To all of this must be added, among other items: (a) the government's growing inability to bail out banks and other fiduciary institutions, who would be in a world of hurt as they foreclosed on bad loans and mortgages without the necessary magnitude of buyers to assume those debts, (b) the growing debt of state, county, and city governments, (c) the hugh personal debts of most consumers, and (d) the rotting physical infrastructure of the country.

"But all we need to do is stimulate the economy," cries the administration's fiscal planner. Wonderful, providing one understands the consequences of encouraging a patient with pneumonia to go run a marathon. That is, it would only ensure a depression, given the unmanageable debt, and there are only three cures for that. The first is sweat equity, where the population gropes and makes do with very little for a period of five to ten years until real wealth catches up with supposed wealth at onset. That's what happened between 1929 and 1939 in this country. The second is triple digit inflation, where the deficit as well as most savings are nullified by way of being rendered worthless. That's what happened in Germany just before the Nazis took over. The third is the refusal of the government to repay its debt, either directly or by confiscatory taxation on the repayment. Economics is often called the "dismal science," but the adjective is mild compared to those that describe the consequences of ignoring fiscal realities.

All this would be bad enough, but the government's entrenched plan to redistribute wealth to the poor and the indigent compounds the difficulties. For starters, the old argument that the tax load imposed on the poor is too heavy is moot. Except for a single individuals without dependents, the poor don't pay taxes anymore. On the contrary, these individuals get an unearned refund plus an enormous range of benefits from the welfare cafeteria. For example, a couple with two children who earned $14,000 in 1991 (well above the poverty line) would owe no federal income tax (on that income) and in addition would receive a basic earned income tax credit of $898 and a health insurance credit of $312. That would compensate for the FICA (Social Security) tax of $1071 and leave a cash credit of $127 to boot, plus the cash value gained from food stamps (which would likely be in the range of $700 to $900).[2] Table A-2 provides more data by income increments of $2,000.

Additionally, lower income earners are now entitled to much higher benefits in proportion to the their FICA tax (which is subsidized to boot) than

---

Table A-2. Net Taxes for Low Income Consumer Units

This table lists federal income and Social Security (FICA) tax liability by increments of gross income, including offsets from the basic earned income credit and the health insurance credit. It does not include the value of food stamps, Medicaid, aid for dependent children (ADC), or other forms of welfare. However, except for food stamps, welfare benefits tend to be cut off at low income levels.

Gross Income	Individual No Dependents	Head of Household One Child	Married Couple Two Children
$2,000	$153	$296 credit	$308 credit
4,000	306	597 credit	621 credit
6,000	525	898 credit	935 credit
8,000	978	1,008 credit	1,051 credit
10,000	1,429	752 credit	898 credit
12,000	1,882	182 credit	625 credit
---- poverty line ------			
14,000	2,335	605	127 credit
16,000	2,788	1,370	600
18,000	3,241	2,148	1,384
20,000	3,694	2,925	2,169

Source: Compiled from tables in *Your Federal Income Tax* [1991] IRS Publication 17.

higher income earners. If you are curious why tables on Social Security entitlements indexed to average earnings are no longer published, seek no further. The attempt to disguise this shift of benefits has been very successful. Moreover, the value of Social Security benefits for higher income earners is reduced by taxation and in some cases by earned income set-offs up through the age of 70. Finally, the wages that can be taxed for Social Security increase significantly each year.

The point to all of this is that the federal government has little to show for this massive welfare, except perhaps a doubling or tripling of the number of illegitimate births. Moreover, this transfer has been primarily at the expense of the so-called "middle class." Tax rates for the wealthy have fallen from a top rate of 70 percent circa 1960 to 31 percent today, although individuals in this bracket, plus the largest 1000 corporations, still pay the lion's share of federal revenues.

Increased subsidization of the poor for the cost of health care needs would only intensify this redistribution of wealth at the price of further weakening the buying power of the middle class. And it is that buying power that sustains the economy. The wealthy, for the most part, don't spend money; they invest it. For every Mercedes on the road, there is twenty times that value invested in stock, bonds and certificates. Unfortunately, those investments lose value when the purchasing capacity of the large middle class implodes, which thus accelerates the decline and fall of the economy. In short, while the health care needs of the poor should be met, the country is no longer in a position to do it without inviting economic disaster, at least not if the standard practice of throwing money at problems continues.

APPENDIX B.

NOTES ON FOREIGN HEALTH CARE SYSTEMS

Similitudes carry with them but very small force of argument,
unless they be in exact agreement with that which is compared.
- John Eachard, 1670

There are many lessons to be learned from foreign health care systems, providing that: (a) the vast differences between the United States and the country being studied are considered, and (b) the negatives are given equal billing with the positives. The one point, however, that does stand out is that no one else seems to be paying as much for health care as this country. In 1987, the U.S. spent 11.2 percent of its GDP on health care, while Canada, Germany, Sweden, and The Netherlands only spent between 8.2 and 9.0 percent.[1] Switzerland got by on 7.7 percent, Japan on 6.8 percent, and the United Kingdom on a mere 6.1 percent. Moreover, health care for low income families and the indigent has been more readily available in every case.

However, this differential stems from three factors, none of which are applicable, or are no longer applicable to the United States. First, with two exceptions, the population and geographical area of all of the countries cited is a small fraction of America's. Sweden, whose system is touted the loudest, has 4 percent of the U.S. land mass and 3.5 percent of its population. For the exceptions, Canada is larger in size but has only a tenth of the population and most of that is concentrated in a one-hundred mile band running along the border, while Japan's population is roughly half that of the U.S. but concentrated in one twenty-fifth the land mass.

There are those who argue that size and population are not significant factors; what works on a small scale can be adapted to work on a large scale. If that were true, then countries with large populations who have tried national health care systems should be doing equally well. Those countries, other than Japan at 124 million, are China (1,134 billion), India (853 million), the former Soviet Union (290 million), Indonesia (181 million), Brazil (150 million), Nigeria (120 million), Pakistan (181 million), and Bangladesh (113 million).[2]

None of them provide health care that remotely compares with the quality and quantity available in the U.S., and those eight countries have over half of the entire world's population. In fact, none of the countries with populations in excess of 100 million, except Japan and the U.S., seem to be doing well at all. They are all poverty stricken to one degree or another.

As to why larger populations are much harder to manage, many theories have been advanced, ranging from excessive span of control to an exponentially rising number of differences among individuals, to the need to win consensus by appealing to an ever declining lowest common denominator. This is no place to review all of those theories, but the facts suggest that the increased difficulties are real and cannot be ignored.

The second difference is that the health care systems in the lower population countries were installed or initiated when costs were much lower and roughly equivalent with the U.S. In some cases, all providers were made employees of the state, and in others fees and costs were rigidly capped (and higher income taxed heavily). Thus even if the U.S. embarked on a similar plan today, the costs would remain higher. The only way to lower them to the 9 percent-of-GDP range would be to cut wages drastically, or alternatively, to ration health care. The former would be unacceptable because it would discriminate against select job classifications, and the latter will likely occur to some degree anyway.

To put the case another way, if the net income (after expenses but before taxes) of physicians was forcefully reduced to the same level as Congressmen, then the health care bill would be reduced by about nine billion dollars. The difference between the average income for physicians and for Congressmen is roughly $22,000 and there are about 420,000 physicians in active practice. The product of those two numbers would equate with about 1.2 percent of the $750 billion price tag of health care. And at that, the government would lose about three billion in taxes it collects on that nine billion.

The third difference is that of cultural disparities between these countries and the United States. Most of them are more inclined to socialism and intense government management of economic affairs. To the extent that a small country has a small homogenous population, this approach will find greater acceptance among the electorate. It doesn't sit well with large heterogeneous populations, witness the recent breakup of the Soviet Union and the simmering discontent in countries that still enforce socialism. China and India come easily to mind.

There is a reason why the United States remains the strongest economic power in the world, and that is the combination of capitalism and democracy. Only Japan gives it any real competition and that country has an unusually strong and almost singular national ethos, sustained in part by the need to support a large population on a small, inhospitable land mass.

Now for the negatives. First, some of these systems are in deep financial trouble, especially Canada. In Ontario, for example, nearly 5,000 hospital jobs and 3,500 beds have been eliminated over the past two years.[3] Similar cutbacks have been made in other provinces, while the free care subsidization fund is drying up. The analysts have finally realized that once a commodity or service is made available regardless of ability to pay, the demand for it will become insatiable, while taxpayers refuse to pay for it. The alternative is to ration health care, which Canada is doing indirectly by way of eliminating providers.

Second, many providers and consumers express intense dissatisfaction with the systems, especially in the United Kingdom (which has the lowest percent-of-GDP cost). The continuous stream of complaints coming out of Great Britain is legendary, and as mentioned, the Canadians are increasingly unhappy. However, this may not true in some of the other countries cited.

Third, as mentioned previously, health services have been intentionally rationed even before funding limitations forced this to happen, especially in the United Kingdom. Older people are routinely denied expensive medical treatments in favor of the young, even when the condition would become terminal in the absence of the treatment, for example a kidney transplant. And for those who are terminally ill, care is strictly limited to control and relief of pain, for example hospices. So-called "aggressive therapy" is out of the question.

Fourth, the systems sometime lead to abuse by way of excessive control over people's private lives. Even the *Reader's Digest* recently carried a story on that trend in Sweden.[4] The Syracuse, New York, case cited earlier in this book (page 24) suggests that this country is not immune to the problem. In sum, then, before health care planners invest one more minute trumpeting the wonders of foreign health care systems, they should take a hard look at the facts as well as the cultural and historical differences. They will find that the good points would be almost impossible to import intact, and even if this could be done, they come packaged with many side-effects.

APPENDIX C.
PROPOSED STUDIES AND SURVEYS

First get your facts, then you can
distort 'em as much as you please.
- Mark Twain

The available data on health care is massive, but it isn't always focused or compiled in the necessary direction. This suggests that a number of special studies or surveys could prove helpful, most of which would be a synthesis of existing, more specialized research and findings. These studies should be done by at least two and preferably three different agencies and the results compared. The more consistent the findings are, the more the weight that should be given to them.

1. Criteria for Closing Excess Hospital Capacity. Of all the elements in this proposal, the forced closing of excess hospital capacity will likely incur the severest negative reaction from providers, and by way of lobbying from Congress itself. This would not be dissimilar to the reactions from the recent Department of Defense base-closing study. Yet if costs are to be contained and a simple per-diem reimbursement formula substituted for the complex entanglements of per-case accounting, there is no other choice.

Unfortunately, the decision-making process could be abused, and even if not, it would still entail difficult and soul-searching trade-offs, not to mention the problems generated by laying off tens of thousands of employees. Then, too, decisions on shutting down entire hospitals versus closing specific wings would be troublesome in many cases. Clearly, this task demands parallel independent studies.

2. Assimilation of Public, VA & Military Hospitals. Under this proposal, the rationale for most public and VA hospitals would change. Funding, per se, would no longer constitute a problem but the general need to maintain existing facilities in urban areas (and the few rural regions) would be as important as ever. Military hospitals, of course, would remain under control of the Department of Defense, but their funding could be integrated with the plan, especially with respect to retirees depending on CHAMPUS and Medicare. Hence this study is necessary to identify the special problems that would arise if these hospitals were integrated for funding purposes under a national plan, or, alternatively, how they would be financed if they remained independent.

3. Potential Sources of Funding. Any national health care plan will be strapped for cash unless every reasonable funding source is tapped. This doesn't mean new taxes on old wineskins. It does mean: (a) identifying sources of funding that would no longer be justified under a national plan, (b) deciding on taxes that could be imposed on products or services that contribute significantly to major health problems, and (c) the effect of various tax or premium formulas on employees. This study should be run in conjunction with the model described in chapter 13, because the coverage and the degree and range of copayments would be the controlling parameters for evaluating the sufficiency or insufficiency of revenues.

4. Providers in Urban Slums and Rural Regions. Before any economic incentives are developed to encourage providers to work in these areas, a definitive survey, or survey of existing regional surveys, is necessary to get a precise handle on the numbers, the geographical distribution, and for slums the hazards involved. It would also include trade-off analyses in special cases on hospitals versus clinics and transportation to outlying hospitals, not to let county and city governments off the hook but where the demographics might warrant that alternative.

5. High-Cost Procedures and Catastrophic Expenses. This study is needed to gauge: (a) the magnitude of the problem in comparison with lesser expenses, and (b) the probability of unleashing even more of them if a national plan is enacted. To the extent this potential exists, how can abuse of it be prevented, especially with respect to doctors attempting to milk the system with terminally ill patients, or hospitals encouraging it as a means of justify expansion of bed capacity? It would be great if providers refrained from doing this, but 25 years of experience with Medicare suggests otherwise.

6. Health Care for the Terminally Ill. Estimates of the percentage of the health care dollar spent during the last six months of life are high and can be verified by careful extrapolation from existing masses of data. What isn't known is how much of that cost is spent on expensive but futile attempts to stop the inexorable progression of death and how much is spent when there is a reasonable chance that life would be prolonged in a way more favorable than a vegetative state. The same analysis should also be applied to those patients who may not be terminal in the formal sense, but who statistically stand almost no chance of surviving more than a few months. This would not be an endearing study, but if an when a national plan is enacted and coverage becomes virtually carte blanc, then sooner or later some hard choices on priorities will have to be made.

7. Pharmaceuticals. Notwithstanding the large number of recent studies in this field, and perhaps because of them, there is a need for a comprehensive survey in precise but readable terms of what drugs are effective, what the generic equivalents are, how effective those equivalents are, the comparative prices of related drugs, the profit margins thereof, the extent to which drugs are prescribed essentially as placebos, the expenditures and extent of promotion by manufacturers, the extent to which some of those promotions are disguised as "objective discussions," the extent of concealment of negative or adverse findings by the industry, and the extent to which multiple prescriptions generate unacceptable toxicity as a side effect. And then put all of it on a computer disk.

8. Conduct and Habits as They Relate to Health. This study would be imperative if a national plan were enacted, because under any such plan health care would come to be regarded as a de facto right. As with any right, it must be adjudicated and that requires an understanding of the responsibilities that go with the right. Hence, conduct and habits that contribute to poor health should diminish the right to, or at least increase the personal cost of, health care, just as criminal conduct can and often does diminishes the right to move about freely for a number of years. It would also provide the basis for proposing disincentive taxes on products that lead to major medical problems.

On a higher level, this study should also examine the implications of the assumptions underwriting psychiatric care, at least those that posit genetic and environmental sources as responsible in part for behavior and mental health. To the extent this is true or assumed to be true is the measure by which the government would be obligated to pay for the medical consequences. But to the extent that personal responsibility is recognized is the extent to which any plan would be able to limit its coverage to more realistic goals.

APPENDIX D.

THE AARP HEALTH CARE PLAN PROPOSAL

Folly is wise in her own eyes.
- Anonymous (dating to 1629)

While this book was being typeset, the American Association of Retired Persons (AARP) published its health care plan proposal (*AARP Bulletin*, March 1992, pp. 1,7,14-15). This proposal is the result of several years of study and is being circulated to members for comment before it becomes the official AARP policy position by April of 1993. The same issue of the Bulletin also announced an increase of member dues from $5.00 to $8.00 per year—a 60 percent increase—which translates into an additional $100 million dollars per year for administration and lobbying. The plan has many similarities with the proposal outlined in this book, but the differences outweigh those similarities. This appendix outlines the principal differences:

• *Scope of Coverage.* Comprehensive, including essentially all forms of long term care and at least some dentistry. And there is no form of rationing whatsoever. All health care services would become carte blanche on demand. And it should be noted that the elderly will benefit the most from the plan as: (a) they are the heaviest users of basic health care services, and (b) the plan includes long-term nursing care.

• *Source of Funding.* In addition to current tax funding for health care, the plan would be financed by: (a) a five percent surtax on corporate income tax. (b) a $600 per year premium for all individuals (supplanting the 1993 Medicare premium of $444 for Medicare enrollees), (c) an eight percent payroll tax on employers, waived for any employer who provides private insurance with equal or better coverage (moot since not one employee in a 50 is covered for long-term nursing care), (d) a three percent flat tax on all income above $15,000 per year ($20,000 for families), (e) a national sales tax on all goods and services except food. housing, and medical care, and (f) a "sin" tax on cigarettes and alcohol.

116

• *Cost Controls.* Except for prohibiting surcharges by providers and placing some limits of drug prices, there are no cost controls and only a few nebulous "national and state budget targets." The fate of Gramm-Rudman should dispel any illusions one may have about the supposed efficacy of budget targets.

The significance of this plan may be stated in the following terms:

• *Orientation.* Although it does provide insurance for everyone, including subsidization of the poor, it is heavily weighted in favor of retirees, especially since it includes long-term care for a mere cost of $156 per year. The overwhelming percentage of the costs would be borne by non-retirees, except for the national "sales tax" on other than food, housing, and medical care. For a family of four making $35,000 per year, assuming 40 percent of what they spend would be subject to the national sales tax and assuming the 8 percent employer tax would be deducted from wages, the cost would be $6350 per year, plus copayments (up to some prescribed limit), plus the existing Medicare tax (1.45 percent of all wages up to $125,000 per year, plus an equal amount from employers).† In some cases, this amount would be offset by the employer's current share of health insurance costs, but many employers do not provide that and would go bankrupt if they had to.

• *Costs.* In the absence of any significant cost control measures, and given the fact that the cost of Medicare increased nearly 3400 percent in its first 25 years, it is not difficult to imagine what will happen to total health care costs. It's a safe bet they would at least double from the current $750 billion per year to 1.5 trillion, exacerbated by the retired fraction of the population increasing (but paying almost nothing for the added coverage), while the working class, which must pay the bill, is shrinking.

Unfortunately, since: (a) almost all providers would become much wealthier under this plan, (b) AARP would have nearly a hundred million dollars per year of new income to lobby for it, and (c) the bulk of its membership would undoubtedly favor it (it being subsidized for them), the plan has an excellent chance of passing. Yet, arguably, given the existing massive federal deficit, it would also drive the country to absolute bankruptcy within five years.

---

† As this went to press, the *AARP Bulletin* (April 1992, p. 11) indicated that readers should choose *between* the special income tax and the national sales tax, not both as stated in the original proposal. This is especially interesting, because until this very year, the Constitution vested the right to initiate tax bills in the U.S. House of Representatives, not AARP.

NOTES

Chapter 1. The Argument

1. A *Profile of Uninsured Americans*, Research Findings 1, National Medical Expenditure Survey, Department of Health & Human services, Publication 89-3443. As of 1987, approximately 37 million Americans were uninsured. The number has risen since then.

2. *State of the Union Address*, January 27, 1992, and subsequent press releases.

3. US Bureau of the Census, *Statistical Abstract of the United States 1991* (111th edition), Washington, DC, 1991, p. 93.

4. *Washington Post*, October 31, 1991, p. A19, and *New York Times*, October 31, 1991, p. A1. The Department of Agriculture is budgeting $28 billion for food stamps in FY 1993.

5. For example, see Louis J. Halle, *Out of Chaos*, and James Gleick, *Chaos: Making a New Science.*

6. *Julius Caesar*, Act IV, Scene 3, lines 218-224.

7. *Iacocca: An Autobiography* (New York: Bantam Books, 1984), pp. 55-56.

8. Samuel Eliot Morison, *The Two-Ocean War* (Boston: Little, Brown and Company, 1963), pp. 146-163. Spruance sunk three and severely disabled the fourth.

Chapter 2. Factors

1. *Statistical Abstract of the United States 1991*, p. 106.

2. *Socioeconomic Characteristics of Medical Practice 1990/1991*, American Medical Association Center for Health Policy Research, pp. 11,152.

3. *AARP Bulletin*, American Association of Retired Persons, February 1992, pp. 1,4.

4. James L. Payne, "Why Congress Can't Kick the Tax and Spending Habit," *Imprimis* (Hillsdale College, Michigan), May 1991, p.2. Mr. Payne subsequently published a book *The Culture of Spending*, which documents the claim.

5. For example, see *Statistical Abstract of the United States 1991*, p. 124. In 1985, 37.5% of the population admitted to having five or more drinks in one day at least once during the year, 30.1% smoked regularly, and 13% were more than 30 percent overweight.

6. "Take the Money and Shut Up," *Newsweek*, January 20, 1992, p. 55.

Chapter 3. Ethics versus Economics

1. *The Rise of American Civilization* (1927). Charles Beard's seminal book on this matter was *An Economic Interpretation of the Constitution of the United States* (1913).

2. F.W. Winterbotham, *The Ultra Secret* (New York, Dell Publishing Co., Inc, 1974), pp. 94-95. This point will not be found in Churchill's own books because he died before the security classification on breaking the Enigma code was lifted, although he did write about the bombings *(Memoirs of the Second World War,* Houghton Mifflin, pp. 378, 404). More than 400 people were killed in the raid.

3. "Not Enough for All," *Newsweek,* May 14, 1990, p. 53.

4. *Modern Maturity,* April-May 1991, p. 7.

Chapter 4. Ethical Centers of Gravity

1. Harry G. Summers, Jr., *On Strategy: The Vietnam War in Context* (Carlisle Barracks, Pennsylvania: Strategic Studies Institute, 1981), pp. 59-66.

2. John O'Brian, "County Defends Splitting Tot-Mom," *Post Standard* [Syracuse, NY], January 18, 1992. I discussed this case with the city editor of that paper on February 26, 1992, who confirmed the details and indicated that Ms. Perrigo's attorney, Ralph Cognetti, was filing suit against the health department, asking for punitive damages. The story has been circulated nationally by the Associated Press (byline Lisa Levitt Ryckman).

3. The case was *Schenck v. United States,* 249 U.S. 47 (1919).

4. See note 3 for chapter 2.

Chapter 5. Economic Centers of Gravity

1. *Statistical Abstract of the United States 1991,* p. 93.

2. Associated Press release, October 10, 1990, Washington, DC.

3. *New York Times,* February 4, 1992, p. A10.

4. See also "Hidden Truth about Hospital Bills, " in *Health,* March-April 1991, condensed in *Reader's Digest,* July 1991.

5. *New York Times,* November 24, 1991, p. A1.

6. Gregg Easterbrook, "The Revolution in Medicine," *Newsweek,* January 26, 1987, pp. 40-68. This may be the single best article ever written on the developing health care crisis.

Chapter 6. Strawman

1. Ironically, the fact that Medicare and CHAMPUS are often jointly administered by the same regional agency was a major influence in formulating the model proposed in the book.

Chapter 7. Ancillaries

1. *Statistical Abstract of the United States 1991*, p. 93. As shown in the table on page 2 of this book, Medicare expenses rose from 7.6 billion to 240.8 billion dollars, an increase of roughly 3400 percent.

2. *New York Times*, June 2, 1991, pp. A1,30

3. Charles B. Clayman, MD, editor, *Encyclopedia of Medicine*, American Medical Association (New York: Random House, 1989), p. 716.

4. Peter Gott, MD, "The Danger of Chiropractic Care," February 19, 1992. The column is widely syndicated.

5. *Encyclopedia of Medicine*, p. 270.

6. *Ibid.*, p. 755.

7. "Pushing Drugs to Doctors," *Consumer Reports*, February 1992, pp. 87-94, and "Miracle Drugs or Media Drugs," March 1992, pp. 142-146.

8. "An Empty Promise to the Elderly?" *Consumer Reports*, June 1991, p. 435, citing data from the Health Care Financing Administration.

Chapter 8. Mental Health Care

1. For example, see A. H. Maslow, "Self Actualizing People," in G.B. Levitas, editor, *The World of Psychology*, volume II (New York, George Braziller, 1963), pp. 527-556.

2. *Health, United States 1990*, DHHS Publication 91-1232, National Center for Health Statistics, (Hyattsville, Maryland: Public Health Service, 1991), p. 51.

3. Franz G. Alexander and Sheldon T. Selesnick, *The History of Psychiatry* (New York: Harper & Row, Publishers, 1966), p. 14.

4. For example see Karl Menninger, *Love Against Hate* (1942) and *Theory of Psychoanalytic Technique* (1958). Also see M. Scott Peck, *The Road Less Traveled.*

Chapter 9. Emotionally-Charged Issues

1. Bill Moyers, *A World of Ideas* (New York: Doubleday, 1989), p. 124.

2. "Health Reform Gridlock? Americans Still Want It Both Ways," *AARP Bulletin*, January 1992, p. 1.

Chapter 10. Automation-Based Issues

1. "Data Bank: Public Safeguard or Blacklist?" *Medical World News*, November 1991, pp. 22-23.

2. *Datapro Reports on Document Imaging Systems*, Datapro Research, Delran, New Jersey. The Association for Image and Information Management, Silver Spring, Maryland, maintains a library of more than 20,000 references, more than half of which cover image processing.

3. *Final Report: Files Archival Image Storage and Retrieval (FAISR)*, September 26, 1988, and Document Processing System, May 7, 1990. The

Request for Proposals (RFP) for the pilot installation at the Austin, Texas, regional office was issued in mid 1991.

4. James L. Cash, et al., *Corporate Information Systems Management*, 2nd edition (Homewood, Illinois: Irwin, 1988), pp. 146-162. This is the principal automation text used at the Harvard Graduate School of Business.

5. The system, limited to diagnosing heart attacks, was developed by Dr. William Baxt of the University of California, San Diego. It was tested on 331 emergency room patients, and apparently will be further tested on a much larger number. The story was circulated nationwide, circa December 1, 1991.

Chapter 11. Infrastructure

1. "Health Care: Cutting Through the Gobbledygook," *Newsweek*, February 3, 1992, p. 24.

2. A substantial number of retirees are not covered by Social Security, but most of them are drawing pensions, especially civil service retirees, and are covered by other health insurance plans.

3. Holy Family Center, which is an arm of Carondelet Health Services (CHS). CHS owns two non-profit hospitals in Tucson (St. Mary's and St. Joseph's), one in Nogales, Arizona, and manages a number of other programs.

4. "An Empty Promise to the Elderly?" *Consumer Reports*, June 1991, pp. 427-428.

Chapter 12. Organization and Responsibilities

1. *Statistical Abstract of the United States 1991*, pp. 18-22.

2. *Black's Law Dictionary*, 4th edition (St. Paul, Minn.: West Publishing Co., 1951), p. 788. The definition is from Brainerd Dispatch Newspaper Co. v. Crow Wing County, 196 Minn. 194, 264 N.W. 779,780.

3. See note 2 for chapter 7.

Chapter 13. Development

1. I learned this by chance when I encountered Mrs. James Miller in a computer store in Arlington, Virginia in 1986. She wanted to buy a computer similar to her husband's but wasn't sure which of two versions to choose. I recommended that she try her husband's first. She replied she could not do that because he kept the national budget on it.

2. This technique would appear to create a circular reference, which is difficult to manage, but it is possible to keep the two computational paths separate.

3. For example, see Department of Defense Directive 5000.29 and Standard 2167.

Chapter 14. Perspective

1. *Iacocca: An Autobiography*, pp. 340-354. See also his Newsweek "My Turn" editorial "Let's End the Poltoonery," April 16, 1990, p. 10, which was a self-admitted reprise to an earlier "My Turn" editorial.

2. *The Republic*, Book VII.

Appendix A. Federal Debt Projections

1. *Bureau of Labor Statistics News*, USDL Publication 90-616, November 11, 1990. See Table 1 "Quintiles of Income before Taxes."

2. Computations are based on *Your Federal Income Tax [1991]*, Publication 17, Department of the Treasury, Internal Revenue Service.

Appendix B. Notes of Foreign Health Care Systems

1. *Source Book of Health Insurance Data 1990*, Health Insurers of America Association, 1991, citing data from the Organization for Economic Cooperation and Development.

2. Population data taken from *1991 Britannica Book of the Year, World Data Section*, pp. 746-751.

3. *New York Times*, November 24, 1991, p. C1.

4. D. Moller, "The Nation that Tried to Buy Happiness," *Reader's Digest*, September, 1991, pp. 100-104.